AF304933

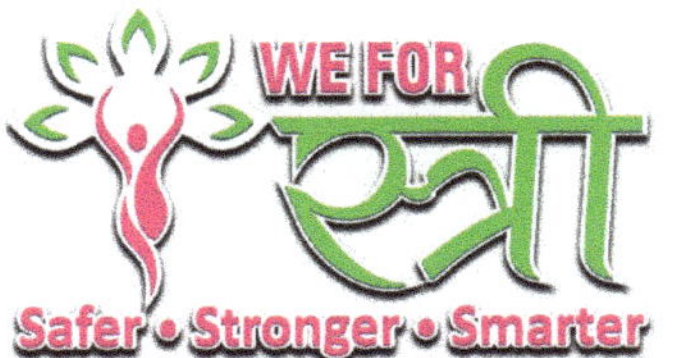
WE FOR
स्त्री
Safer • Stronger • Smarter

FOGSI Focus
Use of Adjuvants in
INFERTILITY

Series Editor

Nandita Palshetkar
MD FCPS FICOG FRCOG (UK)
President FOGSI 2019
Scientific Director, Bloom IVF
Professor
Department of Obstetrics and Gynecology
Dr DY Patil Medical College, Hospital and Research Center
Navi Mumbai, Maharashtra, India

Editors

Sunita Tandulwadkar
MD (Obstetrics and Gynecology) FICS (Gyne-Endoscopy) FICOG
Head, Department of Obstetrics and Gynecology, Ruby Hall Clinic, Pune, Maharashtra, India
Chief, Ruby Hall IVF and Endoscopy Center, Pune
Director, Solo Clinic, Center of Excellence Infertility and Endoscopy
Founder and Medical Advisor, Solo Stem Cells, Stem Cells Research and Application Center, Pune
Chief, IVF and Endoscopy Department, Dr DY Patil Medical College, Pune, Maharashtra
Co-Founder, Solo Research Foundation—Sponsor a Birth
President, IAGE (2019–2020)
Chairperson, Maharashtra Chapter ISAR (2018–2020)
2nd Vice President, Indian Society of Assisted Reproduction (ISAR) (2020–21)
Founder Secretary, Maharashtra Chapter ISAR
Vice-President, West Zone FOGSI (2017)
Chairperson, FOGSI Infertility Committee (2011–2013)
Elected Board Member, International Society of Gynecological Endoscopist (ISGE) (2013–2017)
Advisor and Reviewer, Journal of Human Reproductive Sciences

Madhuri Patil
MD DGO FCPS DFP FICOG (Mum)
Clinical Director, Dr Patil's Fertility and Endoscopy Clinic, Bengaluru, Karnataka, India
Editor-in-Chief, Journal of Human Reproductive Sciences
Associate Editor, The Onco Fertility Journal
Editorial Board Member, Endocrine Society 2020 and 2021
Founder President, Karnataka Chapter of Indian Society for Assisted Reproduction
Vice-President and Founder Member, Fertility Preservation Society (India)
Vice-President and Founder Member, PCOS Society (India)

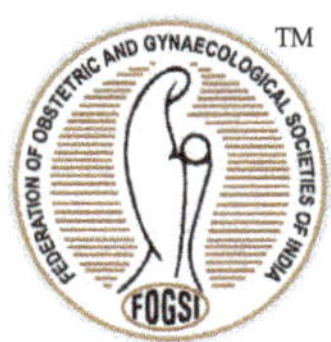

Federation of Obstetric and Gynaecological Societies of India (FOGSI)

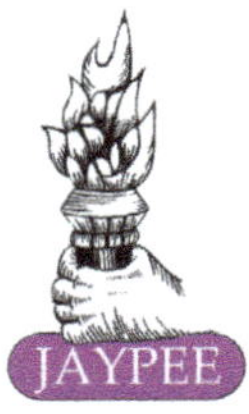

JAYPEE BROTHERS MEDICAL PUBLISHERS
The Health Sciences Publisher
New Delhi | London

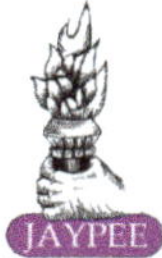 **Jaypee Brothers Medical Publishers (P) Ltd**

Headquarters
Jaypee Brothers Medical Publishers (P) Ltd
4838/24, Ansari Road, Daryaganj
New Delhi 110 002, India
Phone: +91-11-43574357
Fax: +91-11-43574314
E-mail: jaypee@jaypeebrothers.com

Overseas Office
JP Medical Ltd
83 Victoria Street, London
SW1H 0HW (UK)
Phone: +44 20 3170 8910
Fax: +44 (0)20 3008 6180
E-mail: info@jpmedpub.com

Website: www.jaypeebrothers.com
Website: www.jaypeedigital.com

FOGSI Focus Use of Adjuvants in Infertility

First Edition: **2021**

ISBN 978-93-89587-97-5

Contributors

Ameet S Patki
Medical Director, Fertility Associates
Mumbai, Maharashtra, India
Hon Associate Professor
K J Somaiya Medical College and Hospital
Mumbai, Maharashtra, India
Consultant
Khar Hinduja Hospital and Surya Group of Hospital
Mumbai, Maharashtra
Past President, MOGS, 2014–15
Chair, West Zone RCOG, 2015–19
2nd Vice President, ISAR, 2019–20
General Secretary Maharashtra ISAR

Bhavana Mittal
Director, IVF Specialist
Shivam IVF and Infertility Center
Max Superspeciality Hospital
New Delhi, India

Dimple Atul Desai
Embryologist
DPU IVF and Endoscopy Center
Pune, Maharashtra, India

Gautam Khastgir
Director
BIRTH Fertility Clinic
Kolkata, West Bengal, India

Madhuri Patil
Clinical Director, Dr Patil's Fertility and Endoscopy Clinic
Bengaluru, Karnataka, India
Editor-in-Chief, Journal of Human Reproductive Sciences
Associate Editor, The Onco Fertility Journal
Editorial Board Member, Endocrine Society 2020 and 2021
Founder President, Karnataka Chapter of Indian Society for
Assisted Reproduction
Vice-President and Founder Member, Fertility Preservation
Society (India)
Vice-President and Founder Member, PCOS Society (India)

Mayoukh Kumar Chakraborty
Consultant in Gynecology, Obstetrics and Reproductive Medicine
BIRTH Fertility Clinic
Kolkata, West Bengal, India

N Sanjeeva Reddy
Professor and Head
Department of Reproductive Medicine and Surgery
Sri Ramachandra Institute of Higher Education and
Research
Chennai, Tamil Nadu, India

Radha Vembu
Associate Professor
Sri Ramachandra Institute of Higher Education and
Research
Chennai, Tamil Nadu, India

Ritu Hinduja
Senior Consultant Fertility Specialist
Nova IVF
Mumbai, Maharashtra, India
Member of Managing Committee, Indian Society of Assisted
Reproduction

Rohan Krishnakumar
ART and Endoscopic Consultant Gynecologist-Obstetrician
J K Women Hospital
Thane, Maharashtra

Seema Pandey
President, Azamgarh Obs Gyn Society
Managing Committee Member, ISAR (2018–20)
Secretary, UP ISPAT (2018)

S Krishnakumar
Endoscopic Surgeon, Gynecologist, Infertility Specialist
JK Women Hospital
Thane, Maharashtra, India

Sonal Sagar Vaidya
Chief Embryologist
ISAR, ACE, IFS, ESHRE
Ruby Hall Clinic
Grant Medical Foundation
Pune, Maharashtra, India

Sujata Kar
Consultant Gynecologist
Kar Clinic and Hospital Pvt Ltd
Bhubaneswar, Odisha, India

Sunita Tandulwadkar
Head, Department of Obstetrics and Gynecology, Ruby Hall Clinic, Pune, Maharashtra, India
Chief, Ruby Hall IVF and Endoscopy Center, Pune
Director, Solo Clinic, Center of Excellence Infertility and Endoscopy
Founder and Medical Advisor, Solo Stem Cells, Stem Cells Research and Application Center, Pune
Chief, IVF and Endoscopy Department, Dr DY Patil Medical College, Pune, Maharashtra
Co-Founder, Solo Research Foundation—Sponsor a Birth
President, IAGE (2019–2020)
Chairperson, Maharashtra Chapter ISAR (2018–2020)
2nd Vice President, Indian Society of Assisted Reproduction (ISAR) (2020–21)
Founder Secretary, Maharashtra Chapter ISAR
Vice-President, West Zone FOGSI (2017)
Chairperson, FOGSI Infertility Committee (2011–2013)
Elected Board Member, International Society of Gynecological Endoscopist (ISGE) (2013–2017)
Advisor and Reviewer, Journal of Human Reproductive Sciences

Swati Sandipan Ingale
Senior Embryologist
ISAR , ACE, IFS, ESHRE
Ruby Hall Clinic, Grant Medical Foundation
Pune, Maharashtra, India

Teena Trivedi Desai
Consulting Obstetrician Gynecologist
Aviva Fertility Clinic
Mumbai, Maharashtra, India

President's Message

It gives me great pleasure to know that the *FOGSI Focus Use of Adjuvants in Infertility* is ready for release. The aim of this FOGSI Focus is to highlight a new emerging frontier in the area of pharmacotherapy, viz. the role of nutraceuticals, medical nutrition therapy and other medications to improve success rates in our field.

The chapters have been written by eminent experts in research and therapy areas including senior FOGSIans and faculty who are in teaching positions throughout the country. I hope this FOGSI Focus will help to improve your understanding of the role of antioxidants, micronutrients, reactive oxygen species, the scientific theories behind medical nutrition therapy and the growing evidence for adjuvant therapies.

The Presidential theme for my FOGSI year 2019 is "We for Stree—Safer, Stronger, Smarter". During the year, we will attempt to focus on academic, social and community health initiatives aimed at improving the profile of women in India. I urge every single one of you to unite and stand with us and contribute to a series of initiatives which will refocus our contributions not only toward the health of Indian women, but also their social, financial and educational upliftment as well.

FOGSI is committed to delivering continuing medical education programs and also has a raft of initiatives to help women from poor socioeconomic areas receive appropriate care through our social and community healthcare initiatives, e.g., the FOGSI Saving Mothers Initiative. The FOGSI Manyata project also aims to bring a certain minimum standard of care to the women of India via accreditation and training of private nursing homes and healthcare personnel.

I congratulate the Editors of the book Dr Sunita Tandulwadkar and Madhuri Patil for their effort in helping to publish this FOGSI Focus and hope that it adds a new dimension in your practical approach to prescribing.

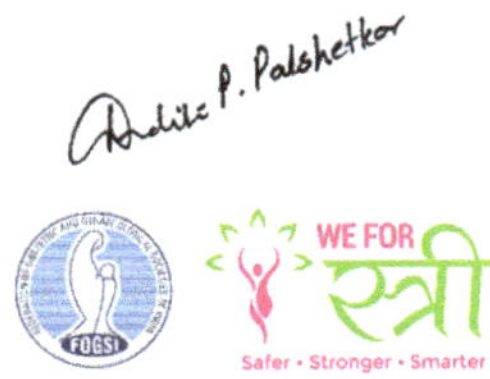

Nandita Palshetkar MD FCPS FICOG
President, FOGSI (2019)
President, IAGE (2017–18)
Chairperson, MSR (2017–18)
Vice President, AMOGS (2016–18)
Past President, MOGS (2016–17)

Preface

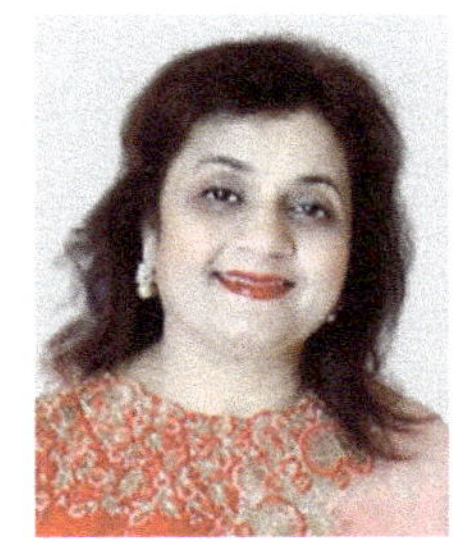

Sunita Tandulwadkar

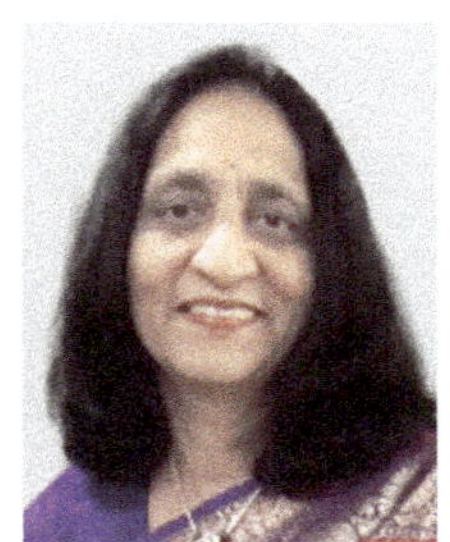

Madhuri Patil

The last two decade has witnessed a striking progress in assisted reproductive technology (ART). There has also been a significant increase in the success rate of ART due to the introduction of adjuvant therapy in clinical practice, novel technologies and improved embryo culture systems. It is important that all ART clinicians keep abreast with all the newer tests, drugs, techniques and technology to implement them in their practice and provide optimal care to their patients.

This book brings fresh insights into the adjuvant therapy that can be used in clinical practice. It also provides up-to-date and practical information on the adjuvants that can be used in the laboratory management of subfertility. Every chapter lay stress on current advances in the potential strategies of various therapeutic options available to improve the management of the sub-fertile couple. Most of these adjuvants have a controversial evidence and this has been covered very well in all the chapters. This will enable each clinician depending on his/her practice conditions to adapt these newer techniques and technologies.

The preparation of this book was driven by a desire of our dear FOGSI president, Dr Nandita Palshetkar (2019) to provide a hands-on practical guide on the various add on treatments in assisted reproduction that would be accessible to those practising in this field. The contributing authors include nationally renowned clinicians and scientists actively involved in the field of reproductive medicine. We are most grateful to all who have made the publication of this "FOGSI Focus" possible.

We hope that you will enjoy reading this ready reckoner on adjuvants in ART as much as we did editing it.

Happy Reading!

Acknowledgments

We thank Nandita Palshetkar, President FOGSI (2019) for giving us the opportunity to publish the *FOGSI Focus Use of Adjuvants in Infertility*. We are extremely thankful to each and every author who has contributed to this edition of the FOGSI Focus. We are especially thankful to Shri Jitendar P Vij (Group Chairman), Mr Ankit Vij (Managing Director), Mr MS Mani (Group President), Ms Chetna Malhotra Vohra (Associate Director—Content Strategy), Ms Pooja Bhandari (Production Head), Ms Kritika Dua (Development Editor) and the publishing staff at M/s Jaypee Brothers Medical Publishers (P) Ltd, New Delhi, India, for their work in completing this book successfully.

Contents

Rational for Additional Therapy in In Vitro Fertilization

Bhavana Mittal

INTRODUCTION

The problem of infertility is at a rise. The treatments for infertility are, however, bound by a limited success rate. Since "necessity is the mother of invention", assisted reproductive technology (ART) is a rapidly evolving field of medicine. Newer drugs and technologies are being tried to improve the result of the procedure. But only a few of them are actually beneficial, safe, and cost effective.

PHARMACOLOGICAL ADJUVANTS

Dehydroepiandrosterone

Dehydroepiandrosterone (DHEA) is a food supplement in many countries. Its mechanism of action in women with decreased ovarian reserve is:

- To increase the production of insulin-like growth factor 1 and estradiol in granulose cells
- To act as a precursor of androstenedione and testosterone in theca cells.

Thereby it improves the follicular function.

In women with normal ovarian reserve, DHEA has not demonstrated any benefit.[1]

In women with diminished ovarian reserve, one meta-analysis has shown improvement in clinical pregnancy rate.[2] A Cochrane review on the same subject, showed a higher pregnancy rate and live birth rate but the benefit was not obvious when studies with high risk of performance bias were excluded.[3]

Side-effects noted with use of long-term DHEA are minor androgenic effects but no long-term risks are seen.

At present, routine DHEA supplementation cannot be recommended in absence of good quality evidence.

Antioxidants Including CoenzymeQ10

Coenzyme Q10 (CoQ10) has been proposed to rejuvenate mitochondrial energy stores in granulosa cells.[4] CoQ10 supplementation has been proposed to defer ovarian aging.[5]

There are only few clinical trials on the application of CoQ10 in assisted reproduction. One randomized controlled trial (RCT) found no improvement in clinical pregnancy rate on use of CoQ10 in a dose of 600 mg daily in *in vitro* fertilization (IVF)/intracytoplasmic sperm injection (ICSI) patients between the age of 35 years and 43 years.[6]

Serious side effects are noted with the use of CoQ10.

CoQ10 cannot be recommended for all poor responders without further evidence.

Growth Hormone

Growth hormone (GH) increases the insulin-like growth factor 1 (IGF-1) level in follicles which potentiates follicle-stimulating hormone (FSH) action on granulosa cells, increases estradiol production and oocyte maturation.

Growth hormone used in a dose of 8–24 IU/day and given daily or alternate day has found to improve live birth rate in poor responders.[7] Low dose (0.5 IU/day) of GH is also sufficient to improve live birth rate in poor responders.[8] A Cochrane review of 10 RCTs showed higher clinical pregnancy rate (CPR) and live birth rate (LBR) when GH was added in women suspected of having low ovarian reserve.[9]

No benefit has been found in the use of GH in normal responders. Also, use of GH is seen in gonadotropin-releasing hormone (GnRH) agonist and not antagonist cycle.[10,11]

Overall, the use of GH as an adjuvant remains inconclusive.

Immune Therapy

The rationale behind immune therapy is maternal immunomodulation around implantation window. Natural killer cells, cytokines, tumor necrosis factor alpha (TNFα), growth factors, and balance between Th1 and Th2 cells are important factors at this time.

However, there are no RCTs on the subject. Also, this treatment can result in some serious side effects and is expensive. At present, immune therapy cannot be offered due to lack of proper evidence, cost, and potential side effects.

Artificial Oocyte Activation

Calcium ionophore releases calcium ions around ooplasm after sperm–oocyte fusion. This can enhance fertilization rate and has been proposed to be beneficial in women with previous ICSI cycle with total failed fertilization.

RCTs in women with reduced ovarian reserve[12] and male infertility[13] did not find any advantage of this intervention. Another systemic review[14] also could not prove any benefit of this treatment.

There is insufficient safety data. At present, this intervention cannot be recommended.

Corticosteroids

Drugs like prednisolone and dexamethasone have been used for immunomodulation at the time of implantation by suppressing natural killer (NK) cells and maintaining cytokines and growth factors.

Use of prednisolone in women with increased NK cells has shown to improve IVF outcome.[15] A significant benefit of prednisolone and heparin has been found in women with unexplained recurrent implantation failure (RIF).[16,17]

Dan et al.[18] found benefit of prednisolone in idiopathic recurrent miscarriage (RM) in terms of increased LBR and reduced miscarriage rate. Short-term use of corticosteroids is not associated with many risks. Currently, prednisolone can be offered in selected patients.

Heparin

Low molecular weight heparin inhibits clotting factor Xa and has been used to prevent microthrombi at implantation site. This promotes trophoblast invasion. Significant improvement in LBR has been shown in women with more than 3 recurrent implantation failure[19] and first IVF cycle.[20] A third RCT, however, failed to show such benefit.[21] Risks associated with heparin are bleeding and thrombocytopenia. Heparin treatment is acceptable in women with thrombophilia. In women without thrombophilia, it should be prescribed in selected cases with proper counseling.

Aspirin

Low dose aspirin is an antiplatelet agent, it improves trophoblast invasion and has been used for implantation failure. A Cochrane review did not find benefit of use of aspirin in RMs.[22] In a review on women with congenital thrombophilia, no benefit of addition of aspirin was seen in terms of LBR or miscarriage rate.[23] Therefore, aspirin should be used in selected cases at present.

Uterine Artery Vasodilators

Sildenafil has been used as a nitric oxide donor. This cause vasodilation and improves endometrial blood flow and thickness. Currently, there is not enough evidence to justify the use of vasodilators to improve implantation.

■ TECHNOLOGICAL ADJUVANTS

Intracytoplasmic Sperm Injection

Intracytoplasmic sperm injection has been accepted in cases of:

- Abnormal semen parameters
- Total failed fertilization with standard insemination
- Fertilization of cryopreserved oocytes
- Fertilization of oocytes matured *in vitro*
- Preimplantation genetic diagnosis (PGD) and pre-implantation genetic screening (PGS) cycles

There is not much evidence in support of the same.

Advanced Sperm Selection Techniques

Embryos with good morphology may not be genetically competent.[24]

Morphology has limited value in predicting implantation potential.[25] It is affected by timing and is observer dependent.[26] There is an effort to select the most competent embryos to increase the success of IVF.

Time Lapse Monitoring

Time lapse monitoring (TLM) has the advantage of continuous monitoring, avoids exposure of embryos, reproducibility, and flexibility of laboratory work. Currently, there is not enough evidence in favor of TLM over conventional morphological assessment.[27] Also, there are concerns over UV rays exposure while taking images and cost of procedure. It can be offered in situations like repeated implantation failure.

TABLE 1: Potential role of various adjuvant therapies in IVF practice.

Therapy or medication	Proposed use in IVF	Safety and possible side effects	Efficacy	Evidence
Acupuncture	Increases pregnancy rates	Safe	Limited evidence	Meta-analysis shows possible benefit with pregnancy in IVF patients
Low dose aspirin	To improve implantation and decrease miscarriage rate	No/low risk/mild side-effects	Limited evidence	Insufficient evidence of the benefit in pregnancy rates in IVF patients
Heparin	To improve implantation and decrease miscarriage rate	No/low risk/mild side-effects	Limited evidence	Studies show inconsistent results Overall, no benefit shown in the pregnancy rate of IVF patients
Melatonin	To improve egg and embryo quality	No/low risk/mild side-effects	No evidence	Antioxidant effect on egg and embryo quality being evaluated
Testosterone	To increase egg numbers and quality in poor responders	Moderate risk/moderate side effects	No/limited evidence	Currently being trialed
DHEA	To increase egg numbers and quality in poor responder	Moderate risk/moderate side-effects	No/limited evidence	Limited small trials with variable results
Growth hormone	To increase egg numbers and quality in poor responders	Moderate risk/moderate side-effects	No evidence	Limited small trials with variable results
Corticosteroids	To improve the implantation rate in patients experiencing repeated IVF failure due to immune dysfunction	High risk/serious side-effects	No evidence	Currently no evidence Still under research
Endometrial injury	To improve embryo implantation	No/low risk Mild side-effects	Limited evidence	To date, studies have been too small to draw any conclusion

(IVF: *in vitro* fertilization; DHEA: dehydroepiandrosterone)

Preimplantation Genetic Screening

Use of PGS by fluorescence *in situ* hybridization (FISH) technique has shown lower success rates in RCTs.[28] No effect was seen in good prognosis women.[29] Next generation sequencing (NGS) in PGS is very accurate, reliable and shows 63.8 % CPR per embryo transfer following NGS.[30,31]

Endometrial Injury

Moderate quality of evidence in favor of endometrial scratching has been found in different RCTs.[32-34] However, these studies have been found to be very heterogeneous in methodology.[35] Endometrial scratching can only be recommended in RIF at present.

Embryo Glue

A Cochrane review on the subject demonstrated increased LBR but increased multiple pregnancy rate also.[36] Embryo glue can be used at present only after proper counseling.

Assisted Hatching

Assisted hatching (AH) has not been found beneficial in good prognosis patients.[37] Another Cochrane review found significant improvement in CPR but no difference in LBR with AH.[38] In women with decreased ovarian reserve, AH showed decreased LBR (Butts, 2014).[39] In absence of corroborative evidence, AH cannot be routinely offered.

■ CONCLUSION

Improvement in the result of ART is the need of the hour. However, any new treatment or "adjuvant" should be judged in terms of theoretical basis of benefit, evidence and favor of its use, potential side-effects, and use **(Table 1)**. There should be proper counseling of the patient before the use of such treatment.

■ REFERENCES

1. Yeung T, Chai J, Li R, et al. A double-blind randomised controlled trial on the effect of dehydroepiandrosterone on ovarian reserve markers, ovarian response and number of oocytes in anticipated normal ovarian responders. BJOG. 2016;123(7):1097-105.
2. Li J, Yuan H, Chen Y, et al. A meta-analysis of dehydro-epiandrosterone supplementation among women with diminished ovarian reserve undergoing in vitro fertilization or intracytoplasmic sperm injection. Int J Gynaecol Obstet. 2015;131(3):240-5.
3. Nagels HE, Rishworth JR, Siristatidis CS, et al. Androgens (dehydroepiandrosterone or testosterone) for women under-going assisted reproduction. Cochrane Database Syst Rev. 2015;(11):CD009749.

4. Bentov Y, Casper RF. The aging oocyte—can mitochondrial function be improved? Fertil Steril. 2013;99(1):18-22.

5. Ben-Meir A, Burstein E, Borrego-Alvarez A, et al. Coenzyme Q10 restores oocyte mitochondrial function and fertility during reproductive aging. Aging Cell. 2015;14(5):887-95.

6. Bentov Y, Hannam T, Jurisicova A, et al. Coenzyme Q10 supplementation and oocyte aneuploidy in women undergoing IVF-ICSI treatment. Clin Med Insights Reprod Health. 2014;8:31-6.

7. Kyrou D, Kolibianakis EM, Venetis CA, et al. How to improve the probability of pregnancy in poor responders undergoing in vitro fertilization: a systematic review and meta-analysis. Fertil Steril. 2009;91(3):749-66.

8. Lattes K, Brassesco M, Gomez M, et al. Low-dose growth hormone supplementation increases clinical pregnancy rate in poor responders undergoing in vitro fertilisation. Gynecol Endocrinol. 2015;31(7):565-8.

9. Duffy JM, Ahmad G, Mohiyiddeen L, et al. Growth hormone for in vitro fertilization. Cochrane Database Syst Rev. 2010;(1):CD000099.

10. Eftekhar M, Aflatoonian A, Mohammadian F, et al. Adjuvant growth hormone therapy in antagonist protocol in poor responders undergoing assisted reproductive technology. Arch Gynecol Obstet. 2013;287(5):1017-21.

11. Dakhly DM, Bayoumi YA, Gad Allah SH. Which is the best IVF/ICSI protocol to be used in poor responders receiving growth hormone as an adjuvant treatment? A prospective randomized trial. Gynecol Endocrinol. 2015;32(2):116-9.

12. Caglar Aytac P, Kilicdag EB, Haydardedeoglu B, et al. Can calcium ionophore "use" in patients with diminished ovarian reserve increase fertilization and pregnancy rates? A randomized, controlled study. Fertil Steril. 2015;104(5):1168-74.

13. Eftekhar M, Janati S, Rahsepar M, et al. Effect of oocyte activation with calcium ionophore on ICSI outcomes in teratospermia: A randomized clinical trial. Iran J Reprod Med. 2013;11(11):875-82.

14. Sfontouris IA, Nastri CO, Lima ML, et al. Artificial oocyte activation to improve reproductive outcomes in women with previous fertilization failure: a systematic review and meta-analysis of RCTs. Hum Reprod. 2015;30(8):1831-41.

15. Gomaa MF, Elkholy AG, El-Said MM, et al. Combined oral prednisolone and heparin versus heparin: the effect on peripheral NK cells and clinical outcome in patients with unexplained recurrent miscarriage. A double-blind placebo randomized controlled trial. Arch Gynecol Obstet. 2014;290(4):757-62.

16. Siristatidis C, Chrelias C, Creatsa M, et al. Addition of prednisolone and heparin in patients with failed IVF/ICSI cycles: a preliminary report of a clinical trial. Hum Fertil (Camb). 2013;16(3):207-10.

17. Fawzy M, El-Refaeey AA. Does combined prednisolone and low molecular weight heparin have a role in unexplained implantation failure? Arch Gynecol Obstet. 2014;289(3):677-80.

18. Dan S, Wei W, Yichao S, et al. Effect of prednisolone administration on patients with unexplained recurrent miscarriage and in routine intracytoplasmic sperm injection: A meta-analysis. Am J Reprod Immunol. 2015;74(1):89-97.

19. Potdar N, Gelbaya TA, Konje JC, et al. Adjunct low-molecular weight heparin to improve live birth rate after recurrent implantation failure: a systematic review and meta-analysis. Hum Reprod Update. 2013;19(6):674-84.

20. Akhtar MA, Sur S, Raine-Fenning N, et al. Heparin for assisted reproduction: summary of a Cochrane review. Fertil Steril. 2015;103(1):33-4.

21. Seshadri S, Sunkara SK. Low-molecular-weight-heparin in recurrent implantation failure. Fertil Steril. 2011;95.

22. de Jong PG, Kaandorp S, Di Nisio M, et al. Aspirin and/or heparin for women with unexplained recurrent miscarriage with or without inherited thrombophilia. Cochrane Database Syst Rev. 2014;(7):CD004734.

23. Areia AL, Fonseca E, Areia M, et al. Low-molecular-weight heparin plus aspirin versus aspirin alone in pregnant women with hereditary thrombophilia to improve live birth rate: meta-analysis of randomized controlled trials. Arch Gynecol Obstet. 2015;293(1):81-6.

24. Alfarawati S, Fragouli E, Colls P, et al. The relationship between blastocyst morphology, chromosomal abnormality, and embryo gender. Fertil Steril. 2011;95(2):520-4.

25. Alpha Scientists in Reproductive Medicine and ESHRE Special Interest Group of Embryology. The Istanbul consensus workshop on embryo assessment: proceedings of an expert meeting. Hum Reprod. 2011;26(6):1270-83.

26. Arce JC, Ziebe S, Lundin K, et al. Interobserver agreement and intraobserver reproducibility of embryo quality assessments. Hum Reprod. 2006;21(8):2141-8.

27. Armstrong S, Arroll N, Cree LM, et al. Time-lapse systems for embryo incubation and assessment in assisted reproduction. Cochrane Database Syst Rev. 2015;(2):CD011320.

28. Mastenbroek S, Twisk M, van der Veen F, et al. Preimplantation genetic screening: a systematic review and meta-analysis of RCTs. Hum Reprod Update. 2011;17(4):454-66.

29. Twisk M, Mastenbroek S, van Wely M, et al. Preimplantation genetic screening for abnormal number of chromosomes (aneuploidies) in in vitro fertilisation or intracytoplasmic sperm injection. Cochrane Database Syst Rev. 2006;(1):CD005291.

30. Fiorentino F, Biricik A, Bono S, et al. Development and validation of a next-generation sequencing-based protocol for 24-chromosome aneuploidy screening of embryos. Fertil Steril. 2014;101(5):1375-82.

31. Fiorentino F, Bono S, Biricik A, et al. Application of next-generation sequencing technology for comprehensive aneuploidy screening of blastocysts in clinical preimplantation genetic screening cycles. Hum Reprod. 2014;29(12):2802-13.

32. El-Toukhy T, Sunkara S, Khalaf Y, et al. Local endometrial injury and IVF outcome: a systematic review and meta-analysis. Reprod Biomed Online. 2012;25(4):345-54.

33. Nastri CO, Lensen S, Polanski L, et al. Endometrial injury and reproductive outcomes: there's more to this story than meets the horse's blind eye. Hum Reprod. 2015;30(3):749.

34. Potdar N, Gelbaya T, Nardo LG, et al. Endometrial injury to overcome recurrent embryo implantation failure: a systematic review and meta-analysis. Reprod Biomed Online. 2012;25(6):561-71.

35. Simon C, Bellver J. Scratching beneath 'The Scratching Case': systematic reviews and meta-analyses, the back door for evidence-based medicine. Hum Reprod. 2014;29(8):1618-21.

36. Bontekoe S, Heineman MJ, Johnson N, et al. Adherence compounds in embryo transfer media for assisted reproductive technologies. Cochrane Database Syst Rev. 2014;(2):CD007421.

37. Martins WP, Rocha IA, Ferriani RA, et al. Assisted hatching of human embryos: a systematic review and meta-analysis of randomized controlled trials. Hum Reprod Update. 2011;17(4):438-53.

38. Carney SK, Das S, Blake D, et al. Assisted hatching on assisted conception in vitro fertilisation (IVF) and intracytoplasmic sperm injection (ICSI). Cochrane Database Syst Rev. 2012;12:CD001894.

39. Butts SF, Owen C, Mainigi M, et al. Assisted hatching and intracytoplasmic sperm injection are not associated with improved outcomes in assisted reproduction cycles for diminished ovarian reserve: an analysis of cycles in the United States from 2004 to 2011. Fertil Steril. 2014;102(4):1041-7.

Various Options of Additional Therapy in In Vitro Fertilization with Best Available Evidence for Each Suggested Therapy: An Overview

Madhuri Patil

INTRODUCTION

We need to optimize the results of assisted reproductive technology (ART), as even after 40 years of in vitro fertilization (IVF) treatment and research there is only marginal improvement in implantation and pregnancy rates, though major progress has been made in improving stimulation protocols and fertilization procedures, optimizing embryo culture conditions, and preventing premature luteinization.

Thirty percent of the embryos are lost at preimplantation stage, another 30% are lost after embryos implant but prior to missed period which is detectable by positive beta-human chorionic gonadotropin (hCG) and 10% are lost after the missed period.[1] Disturbance in the embryo–maternal dialog is the major reason for 60% of all pregnancies terminated at end of the peri-implantation period.

As even failure of the first cycle can be devastating, we need to optimize the results after ART and thus comes the role of adjuvants in IVF. Adjuvants are substances or therapies that help and enhance the effect of a drug, treatment, or biologic system.

ADD-ONS IN IN VITRO FERTILIZATION PROGRAM

The add-on or adjuvant therapies could be pharmacological or nonpharmacological agents, surgical procedures, or additional interventions in the IVF laboratory **(Table 1)**.

Before advising these therapies, one must remember that they should be chosen with great care as they are expensive with questionable actual advantage.

Pharmacological Adjuvants

An adjuvant is a substance that enhances the pharmacological effect of a drug.

TABLE 1: Adjuvant therapies in ART.

Adjuvants	Therapies

Pharmacological adjuvants	• To optimize ovarian response
	• *Adjuvants in treatment of poor responders:*
	  – Growth hormone (GH)/GH-releasing factor (GHRF)
	  – Pyridostigmine
	  – DHEA/testosterone
	  – Aspirin
	  – L-arginine
	  – Aromatase inhibitors
	  – Estrogen pretreatment
	  – GCSF
	• *Adjuvants in treatment of PCOS:*
	  – Glucocorticoids—prednisone, methylprednisolone, and dexamethasone
	  – Metformin
	  – Myoinositol
	  – N-acetylcysteine
	  – Melatonin
	  – Vitamin D
	  – Chromium polynicotinate
	• *To optimize ART outcome:*
	  – Antioxidants—coenzyme Q10
	  – Micronutrients
	  – Dopamine agonist
	  – Aspirin
	  – Heparin
	  – Immune therapy
	  – Vasodilators—sildenafil
	  – Calcium ionophores

Nonpharmacological adjuvants	• Acupuncture • Acupressure • Massages • Reiki • Hypnosis

Contd...

Contd...

Adjuvants	Therapies
Surgical adjuvants	• Routine hysteroscopy • Endometrial scratch • Hysteroscopic removal of polyps and submucous myoma, septum • Removal or disconnection of hydrosalpinx • Management of ovarian endometrioma • Laparoscopic ovarian drilling
New technologies	• Advanced sperm selection procedures • Time-lapse embryo monitoring • Preimplantation genetic screening • Assisted hatching • Use of embryo glue

(ART: assisted reproductive technology; DHEA: dehydroepiandrosterone; GCSF: granulocyte colony-stimulating factor; PCOS: polycystic ovary syndrome)

Adjuvants to Enhance In Vitro Fertilization Outcome in Poor Responders

Adjuvants in poor responders can modify the intraovarian environment.

- *Growth hormone (GH)*: GH enhances gonadotropin effects on granulosa cells (GCs) and its action on the liver, increasing insulin-like growth factor-1 (IGF-1) systemically, which in turn will act on the follicle resulting in oocyte maturation and enhanced follicle growth and steroidogenesis.[2] IGF-1 synergizes with follicle-stimulating hormone (FSH) in its effect in inducing GC aromatase activity and also stimulates thecal androgen production, synergizing with luteinizing hormone (LH). Beneficial effect of GH is also seen on the probability of clinical pregnancy rate (CPR) and live birth rate (LBR) in women with decreased ovarian reserve (DOR) and poor responders.[3-6] However, no improvement in LBR was noted in the presence of previous suboptimal response to controlled ovarian stimulation (COS).[5] The most recent publication has shown no statistically significant benefit on CPR, LBR, and ongoing pregnancy rate.[7] The role of GH to treat a woman with a poor response to ovarian stimulation cannot be supported on the basis of the available evidence.[8-10]
- *Growth hormone-releasing factor (GHRF)*: Earlier reports showed that GHRF when given in the dose of 500 µg twice daily enhances gonadotropin-induced steroidogenesis, cyclic adenosine monophosphate (cAMP) formation. It also increases GH and IGF-1 concentration, thus improves the ovarian response to gonadotropins.[11,12] However, a large multicentric, prospective, randomized, double-blind, placebo-controlled trial (196 patients) showed no beneficial effect on the CPR, LBR, and cycle cancelation rate.[12] GHRF also had no beneficial effect on the outcome and had no significant effect on mean number of follicles with a diameter of ≥16 mm, days of stimulation, and total dose of gonadotropin required.[12]

- *Addition of pyridostigmine*: Pyridostigmine is an acetylcholinesterase inhibitor, when given in the dose 120 mg/day orally can increase GH secretion by enhancing the action of acetylcholine.[13] Addition of pyridostigmine does not improve the ongoing pregnancy rate or LBR in poor responders undergoing IVF.[14] However, Chung-Hoon et al. in 1999 reported beneficial effect of pyridostigmine on total dose of gonadotropins (38.4 ampoules vs. 48.3 ampoules), number of oocytes retrieved (5.9 vs. 3.7), and CPR (25.7% vs. 11.4%).[15]

- *Androgens pretreatment*: Androgens increase FSH receptor expression in GCs, stimulating IGF-1, which may have a beneficial effect on the number of small antral follicles and also improve the ovarian sensitivity and responsiveness to FSH.[16-19] Use of transdermal testosterone or dehydroepiandrosterone (DHEA) pretreatment in poor responders undergoing COS for ART is safe and effective way of increasing the intraovarian androgen concentration.[20,21] Androgens decrease the dose of gonadotropin required and duration of stimulation and also increase in the number of cumulus-oocyte complexes (COCs) retrieved.[22] Transdermal testosterone pretreatment at a dose of 10 mg/day for 21 days was associated with decreased duration and total dose of gonadotropin, increased number of COCs retrieved, and an increased CPR (+15%) and LBR (+11%).[22] The same author in 2016 concluded that testosterone did not increase the number of COCs retrieved by >1.5 in poor responders and there was also no increase in LBR.[23]

  - *Dehydroepiandrosterone administration*: Marked heterogeneity of treatment group made a firm conclusion on therapeutic efficacy of DHEA difficult. The rationale for its use is related to decline of DHEA in older women that contributes to the reduced circulating and intraovarian testosterone. Administration of DHEA can have a direct effect on the aging ovary by increasing the pool of follicles up to the preantral stage. It can also reduce apoptosis of the originally recruited follicles and affect the nondysfunctional events happening during meiosis. DHEA can also improve steroidogenesis, since it is a precursor of estradiol and testosterone[24] and may influence ovarian follicular growth by serving as ligands for androgen receptors.[24]

First use of DHEA was reported by Casson PR et al. in 2000[20] in patients aged 35–40 years and having normal FSH concentrations. He concluded that DHEA can augment response to ovulation induction in poor responders with higher number of follicles >15 mm and peak estradiol value, though much difference in the gonadotropin dose was not noted.[25,26] Barad et al., 2007 and Hyman et al., 2010 reported increased oocyte yield (4.4 + 0.5 vs. 3.4 + 0.5; P: 0.05), higher fertilization rate (67% vs. 39%; P: 0.001) and higher embryo grade (3.4 + 0.09 vs. 2.9 + 0.1; P: 0.02), increased pregnancy rate (28.4% vs. 11.9%; P: 0.05), and significantly lower miscarriage rates following DHEA supplementation. Mamas and Mamas, 2009[27] (5 patients) and Sönmezer et al., 2009[28] (19 patients) in addition to the above also reported increased number of metaphase II oocytes (4 + 1.8 vs. 2.1 + 1.8; P: 0.05), increased number of day 3 high quality embryos (1.9 + 0.8 vs. 0.7 + 0.6; P: 0.05), and higher pregnancy rates (47.4% vs. 10.5%; P: 0.01). Wiser et al. also showed a beneficial effect on the LBR.[29]

Dehydroepiandrosterone supplementation also increased anti-Müllerian hormone (AMH) levels in patients with DOR in parallel with the duration of use and increase was more prominent in younger women.[30-34] These women who had an increase in AMH levels were more likely to become pregnant and also showed a lower rate of embryonic aneuploidy in the DHEA group (38.2% vs. 61%) as detected by preimplantation genetic screening (PGS).[33,34] This increase in AMH was not validated by other authors.[35,36] Benefit after DHEA was seen only after it was given for an average of 8.5 weeks.[29] As most these studies which showed benefit were mostly small case series, there were several other studies that showed conflicting results and have suggested large-scale, well-designed confirmatory randomized controlled trials (RCTs) to prove the efficacy of DHEA before it can be recommended for routine use.[22,37-39]

Zhang M et al.,[40] J Assist Reprod Genet, April 2016, concluded based on the limited available evidence that DHEA supplementation seems to improve antral follicle count, AMH, oocyte number, implantation rate, CPR, and LBR in patients with poor ovarian reserve (POR). However, he also suggested further research to clarify the effect of DHEA exposure in ART.

The Cochrane review in 2015 concluded that androgen supplementation prior to ovarian stimulation is not supported by the best available evidence though it may be associated with improved LBR.[41] This review also said that there is insufficient evidence to draw any conclusions about the safety of either androgen. Although some scientific evidence seems to support the use of androgen pretreatment in POR, several authors have recommended further studies for its use.[42,43]

- *Aspirin*: Administration induces a shift from thromboxane A2 to prostacyclin, leading to vasodilatation and increased peripheral blood supply. A meta-analysis to determine the effect of low-dose aspirin versus placebo or no treatment on the likelihood of clinical outcomes in IVF/intracytoplasmic sperm injection (ICSI) cycles was conducted.[44] LBR was reported only in two trials and analytical pooling showed no significant difference [odds ratio (OR): 1.08; 95% confidence interval (CI): 0.83–1.40].[44] Low-dose aspirin did not have any effect in poor responders[45] and in recipients of donated oocytes.[46,47] Another RCT which looked at combination adjuvant therapy with low-dose aspirin and prednisolone concluded that it does not improve uterine blood flow, implantation, and pregnancy rates.[48] They concluded that low doses of acetylsalicylic acid (ASA) and prednisolone are able to improve ovarian responsiveness to gonadotropins in good-prognosis IVF patients, but do not significantly improve uterine blood flow and pregnancy and implantation rates.[48] They also concluded that this combination could be effective in preventing the onset of severe ovarian hyperstimulation syndrome (OHSS) in high-responder patients during IVF.[48] Yet another meta-analytical pooling showed primary increase in clinical pregnancy rates, but more data is necessary to resolve the issue.[49] But this study also concluded that at this point, there is no reason to change clinical management and discontinue the use of aspirin.[49]
- *L-arginine*: Enhanced vascularization appears to be important for follicular selection and maturation in both spontaneous and stimulated IVF cycles. Nitric oxide, formed in vivo from L-arginine, may play a key role in follicular maturation and ovulation.
  Oral L-arginine supplementation in normally responding patients increases follicular recruitment and reduces the duration of pure FSH (pFSH) treatment, but might also have detrimental effects on embryo quality and pregnancy rate.[50]
- *Estrogen pretreatment*: Pretreatment with ethinyl estradiol improves the success rate of ovulation induction with exogenous gonadotropins in patients with DOR.[51] But for this threshold of 15 mIU/mL for FSH should be achieved before starting ovarian stimulation.[51]

- *Colony-stimulating factor*: Prospective study of 30 women, where concomitant administration of colony-stimulating factor-1 (CSF-1) and human menopausal gonadotropin (hMG) improved follicle developments, especially in patients with low serum CSF-1 levels in the early follicular phase.[52] No RCTs still and therefore further large-scale, controlled trials are required to assess the efficacy of CSF-1 as adjuvant therapy for poor responders.
- *Letrozole*: Letrozole cotreatment in a gonadotropin-releasing hormone (GnRH) antagonist protocol in poor responders undergoing ART. Two publications have shown that there is insufficient evidence to recommend use of letrozole (low as well as high dose) as an adjuvant in ART stimulation protocols of poor responder patients.[53,54] One publication by Hakan Yarali[55] has shown the effectiveness of letrozole in an antagonist protocol in poor responders. But he has also suggested that future powerful RCTs delineate the optimum controlled ovarian hyperstimulation (COH) protocol to be used in poor responders.[55]

Adjuvants in Polycystic Ovary Syndrome

It can be used for:

- Treatment of androgen excess—prednisone, methyl-prednisolone, and dexamethasone (DEX).
- Hyperinsulinemia/insulin resistance—metformin, inositol.
- Others—N-acetylcysteine (NAC), melatonin, vitamin D, chromium polynicotinate, and L-methylfolate.
- *Glucocorticoids*: Glucocorticoids have been proposed as a useful adjuvant to both clomiphene citrate (CC) and gonadotropin ovulation induction in women with polycystic ovary syndrome (PCOS) with a therapeutic rationale based on reducing adrenal androgen levels, improving ovulatory function, and reducing resistance to ovulation induction agents.[56,57] Glucocorticoids reduce adrenal androgen production by negative feedback inhibition of adrenocorticotropic hormone production which in turn may reduce total circulating androgen levels by as much as 40%, improving folliculogenesis. While major complications from the adjuvant use of low-dose glucocorticoids are rare, weight gain is a common problem. Other reported side effects include glucose intolerance and osteoporosis. Given possible side effects, their use should remain as a second-line therapy.[56,58]

Dexamethasone is used to treat patients with PCOS who have either adrenal or mixed adrenal and ovarian hyperandrogenism and is given in the dose of 0.25 mg at night from day 2 to 11 of menstrual cycle when undergoing ovulation induction and is supposed to suppress dehydroepiandrosterone sulfate (DHEAS). Aim is to reduce concentration of DHEAS to <400 µg/dL. A study evaluated the effects of short-course administration of DEX combined with CC in CC-resistant patients with PCOS. Eighty-eight percent of the treatment group and 20% of the control group had evidence of ovulation. 46 (40.5%) pregnancies resulted after the combined use of CC and DEX whereas only five (4.2%) women in the control group conceived.[58]

- *Ketoconazole*: Ketoconazole in the dose of 200 mg/day inhibits the key steroidogenic cytochromes with significant reduction in the levels of androstenedione, total and free testosterone.
- *Metformin*: Metformin belongs to the class of biguanides and is the most common drug used as first-line oral therapy for the treatment of type 2 diabetes. Metformin reduces glucose production in the liver, decreases glucose absorption in the intestine, increases insulin secretion in the pancreas, and increases the peripheral glucose uptake in the adipose tissue and muscle.

Anovulatory women with PCOS and who are resistant to CC may be prescribed metformin as a second-line treatment as adjuvant therapy to CC and gonadotropin ovulation induction. It may also be used as an adjuvant therapy to reduce the risk of developing OHSS in PCOS women undergoing GnRH agonist long protocol IVF/ICSI.[59] After initial reports of effectiveness of metformin in 2015, it was recommended not to use it as monotherapy or in combination with CC for primary ovulation induction, as it has not been shown to improve LBRs. It was recommended to be used as an off-label manner to help improve menstrual cycle regularity or hyperandrogenism in women with PCOS who cannot tolerate or have contraindications to combined oral contraceptive pills.[60] Later in 2017, the Cochrane review concluded that metformin may increase the LBR among women undergoing ovulation induction with gonadotropins in both IUI and ART cycles. This review also said that there is insufficient evidence to show an effect of metformin on multiple pregnancy rates and adverse events like OHSS.[61]

In 2017, another Cochrane review[62] looked at the role of insulin sensitizers and concluded that:

- Metformin alone may be beneficial over placebo for LBR, although the quality of evidence was low
- Data on metformin versus CC for LBR is inconclusive and limited by lack of evidence
- Results differed by body mass index (BMI), emphasizing the importance of stratifying results by BMI

- Clomiphene citrate resulted in improvement in CPR and ovulation as compared to metformin alone in obese women with PCOS
- Combined therapy of metformin and CC versus CC alone resulted in improved ovulation rate and CPR, but it is not known whether this translates into increased LBR
- Women taking metformin alone or with combined therapy have no evidence of increased miscarriages or gastrointestinal side effects.

Although there is no current evidence that metformin is teratogenic, when used widely to treat anovulation, then it is possible that rare effects may be unmasked. Metformin therapy therefore needs to be kept under continuing surveillance and adverse outcomes reported.[62]

- *Inositol*: Inositol is a member of the B-complex family of vitamins, but not an essential vitamin and tends to be deficient in women with PCOS. These decreased levels of inositol along with increased urinary clearance of inositol can result in insulin resistance and hyperinsulinemia.[63] Myoinositol increases insulin sensitivity, decreases insulin resistance, improves glucose utilization, decreases free and total testosterone, and restores menstruation and normal ovulation.[64] Myoinositol plays an important role for the signal pathways of cells, particularly in individuals with PCOS. An improved insulin sensitivity may be observed due to the action of myoinositol in PCOS pathway. Several studies indicate that myoinositol is an effective alternative in the treatment of PCOS with no side effects with a standard dosage.[65] Myoinositol has shown beneficial effects on ovarian function and response to ART in women with PCOS as it induces nuclear and cytoplasmic oocyte maturation and promotes embryo development. There is no data available on its effects on pregnancy rate and LBR. In contrast, D-chiro-inositol appears to exert opposite and detrimental effects on the ovary.[66] Further research on larger patient populations is needed to determine whether inositol supplementation, possibly in combination with other drugs, could improve CPR and LBRs in PCOS women undergoing ART.
- *N-acetylcysteine*: NAC as an adjuvant improves insulin sensitivity, decreases androgen level, prevents follicular cohort atresia, and improves quality of cervical mucus. NAC is a safe and well-tolerated adjuvant to CC for induction of ovulation that can improve the ovulation and pregnancy rates in PCOS patients. It may also have some beneficial impacts on endometrial thickness.[67,68]
- *Melatonin*: Melatonin is a hormone of pineal gland, maintains normal circadian rhythms, and governs release of pituitary gonadotropins. Melatonin receptors have been identified in anterior pituitary and ovary also. It is involved in follicular development, ovulation, oocyte maturation, and luteal function. Melatonin deficiency seems to be involved in pathophysiology of PCOS. Melatonin is also a powerful free radical scavenger and has broad-spectrum antioxidant property and has shown to reverse glucose intolerance. Melatonin is taken up into the follicular fluid from the blood and the reactive oxygen species (ROS) produced within the follicles, especially during the ovulation process, was scavenged by melatonin and reduced oxidative stress involved in oocyte maturation and embryo development with improved fertilization and pregnancy rates.[69,70] Despite the antioxidant action of melatonin as per recent meta-analysis, there is no clarity regarding benefit of adding melatonin in all PCOS women.[69,71]
- *Vitamin D*: Vitamin D is a steroid hormone synthesized in the skin by ultraviolet light. Several studies have indicated that most of the women with PCOS are vitamin D deficient. Vitamin D deficiency may be associated with obesity, insulin resistance, and metabolic syndrome, all of which are commonly observed in PCOS and ovulatory dysfunction. In women with PCOS, vitamin D can improve menstrual irregularity, follicular development, and pregnancy rate.[72]
- *Chromium polynicotinate*: Chromium polynicotinate consists of pure niacin-bound chromium binds to niacin and provides a biologically active form of chromium and makes it easier for the body to absorb active component of glucose tolerance factor which is responsible for binding insulin to cell membrane receptor sites, improves insulin sensitivity, and stimulates the metabolism of sugar, fat, and cholesterol. Its deficiency may result in insulin resistance and evidence from clinical studies suggests that low levels of chromium may disrupt glucose and insulin regulation. It is used as an adjuvant therapy for the treatment of anovulation in infertile patients with PCOS.[73]
- *L-methylfolate*: L-methylfolate is a natural, active form of folic acid used at the cellular level for DNA reproduction and the regulation of homocysteine. It reduces homocysteine levels and prevents cardiovascular risk factors associated with PCOS. L-methylfolate, an unmethylated form of folic acid (vitamin B9), is a synthetic form of folate found in nutritional supplements.
- *Coenzyme Q10 (CoQ10)*: CoQ10 seems to be a promising adjuvant to oral ovulatory agents such as CC. It is effective, inexpensive, and safe for stimulating follicular development in CC-resistant PCOS and can be tried successfully before a more complicated treatment such as gonadotropins and laparoscopic ovarian drilling.[74]

Adjuvants that Reduce the Incidence of Ovarian Hyperstimulation Syndrome

Adjuvants that reduce the incidence of OHSS are described in **Table 2**.

Adjuvants Used to Optimize Assisted Reproductive Technology Outcome

- *Immunoglobulins*: The mode of action is far from being fully understood. It may be of use in improving ART outcome in women with raised peripheral natural killer (NK) cells, positive antithyroid antibodies, positive antiphospholipid antibodies, and shared human leukocyte antigens. But studies have shown that intravenous immunoglobulin (IVIg) failed to improve the LBR in couples with repeated unexplained IVF failure.[75] After this, one publication concluded that IVIg treatment significantly increases the LBR in couples with repeated unexplained IVF failure.[76] But one must remember that immunoglobulins can be associated with anaphylaxis, headache, malaise, flushing, fever, nausea, tachycardia, renal failure, aseptic meningitis, thromboembolic events, and hemolytic anemia.[77]

- *Intralipid*: Twenty percent intravenous fat emulsion made up of egg yolks, soya oil, and water are used as a source of fat and calories in parenteral nutrition. It may help to potentiate the immune system and is not expensive and easy to administer. Not used routinely due to lack of evidence.

- *Steroids*: Steroids alter cytokine production, decrease uterine natural killer (uNK) cells, and modulate autoantibodies expression, but no significant difference was seen in the pregnancy rates, LBR, and ongoing pregnancy rate.[78] These findings were limited to the routine use of glucocorticoids and cannot be extrapolated to women with autoantibodies, unexplained infertility, or recurrent implantation failure (RIF).[78]

- *Vasodilators (sildenafil citrate)*: In a quasi-randomized trial, IVF patients failing to attain an embryo transfer (ET) ≥8 mm were administered sildenafil. It was observed that neither endometrial thickness nor blood supply improved after sildenafil therapy.[79]

- *Aspirin*: Administration of aspirin induces a shift from thromboxane A2 to prostacyclin, leading to vasodilatation and increased peripheral blood supply. Aspirin and heparin are beneficial for women with recurrent miscarriage and antiphospholipid (APL) syndrome.[80,81] RCTs to determine the effect of low-dose aspirin versus placebo or no treatment on the likelihood of clinical outcomes in IVF/ICSI cycles with CPR as the primary outcome did not show any statistical difference. Of these RCTs, LBR was reported only in two trials and analytical pooling showed again no significant difference (OR: 1.08; 95% CI: 0.83–1.40).[44] There was another systemic analysis and meta-analysis published in Fertility and Sterility, which also did not support the use of aspirin in IVF or ICSI treatment on the basis of available evidence does not support. They suggested a definitive trial to show improvement in CPRs.[47]

- *Heparin*: Coagulation disorders could interfere with the different stages of embryo implantation.[82] There is a definite benefit of using heparin in patients with recurrent pregnancy failure related to antiphospholipid antibodies (APS) or other thrombophilic disorders.[83] Use of such antithrombolytic therapies in patients with RIF and without thrombophilic disorders is still debatable

TABLE 2: Adjuvants to reduce the incidence of OHSS.

Drugs	Effect	Evidence
Cabergoline	Reduces the effects of VEGF-mediated vascular permeability without compromising IR and PR	Grade A
IV calcium infusion (10 mL of 10% calcium gluconate in 200 mL normal saline)	• On the day of oocyte retrieval and days 1, 2, and 3 after oocyte retrieval can decrease OHSS risk • Increased calcium is postulated to inhibit cAMP-stimulated renin secretion, which decreases angiotensin II synthesis and its subsequent effect on VEGF production	Grade B
Prophylactic albumin administration at OR	Clear benefit from IV albumin at OR by increasing the intravascular osmotic pressure thus preventing occurrence of severe OHSS in high-risk cases (OR: 0.28; 95% CI: 0.11–0.73)	Grade C
Hydroxyethyl starch (HAES)	Significantly increases intravascular volume, therefore raising osmotic pressure. It also inhibits platelet aggregation with beneficial effect in decreasing OHSS	GPP
Immunoglobulin	Severe OHSS is associated with low IgG, IgA gamma globulins and therefore administration of IV gamma globulins reduces the severity	No evidence
Corticosteroids	100 mg IV hydrocortisone after OR and followed orally by methylprednisolone effectively reduces the incidence of severe OHSS	No evidence

(cAMP: cyclic adenosine monophosphate; CI: confidence interval; IgA: immunoglobulin A; IgG: immunoglobulin G; IV: intravenous; OHSS: ovarian hyperstimulation syndrome; OR: odds ratio; VEGF: vascular endothelial growth factor) as no significant effect on increase in implantation and the rate of live birth was observed.[84-89]

- *Antioxidants and micronutrients*: Supplementing diets with mitochondrial nutrients such as CoQ10 and r-alpha-lipoic acid may potentially be beneficial. We are aware that increased oxidative stress can result in altered glucose metabolism, decreased antiglycation defenses, increased mitochondrial dysfunction, and progressive metabolic impairment.

  Substantial evidence has indicated that some physiological processes, from oocyte maturation to fertilization and embryo development, are particularly sensitive to oxidative stress (OS). These processes require antioxidants for balanced function. The additional treatment with micronutrients, starting 3 months before IVF cycles, protects the follicular microenvironment from oxidative stress, thus increasing the number of good quality oocytes recovered at the pickup.[90,91]

Nonpharmacological Adjuvants

- *Acupuncture*: Used in China for centuries to regulate the female reproductive system. Recent popularity in the Western world. There are three potential mechanisms, which increase neurotransmitters, FSH, estradiol, and uterine blood flow. In traditional acupuncture, the needles were inserted in classical meridian points, or contemporary acupuncture in which the needles were inserted in non-meridian or trigger points.

  Figure 1 shows the acupuncture points.
  Acupuncture can be done during ovarian stimulation, at oocyte recovery, before and after ET. Few systemic reviews and meta-analysis have been conducted on its effectiveness as an adjunct treatment and it is not recommended as a routine use procedure.[92]
- *Acupressure*: In acupressure, stimulation of certain points of the body balances the flow of vital energy. Kovárová et al.[93] observed a significant increase in women's self-efficacy after four sessions of treatment with acupuncture. On the other hand, Cheong et al.[94] did not observe any evidence of overall benefit of acupuncture on improving the LBR.

  Figure 2 illustrates the acupressure points.
- *Massage therapy* prior to ET improves implantation, most likely due to reduction in stress as a result of relaxation effect, reduction in uterine contractions, and an enhancement of blood flow in the abdominal region was also noted (Okhowat J et al., 2015).[95]
- *Complementary and alternative medicines (CAMs)— Reiki and Hypnosis*: CAMs are sometimes used to improve the outcomes of fertility treatment and/or mental health during fertility treatment. Overall, the

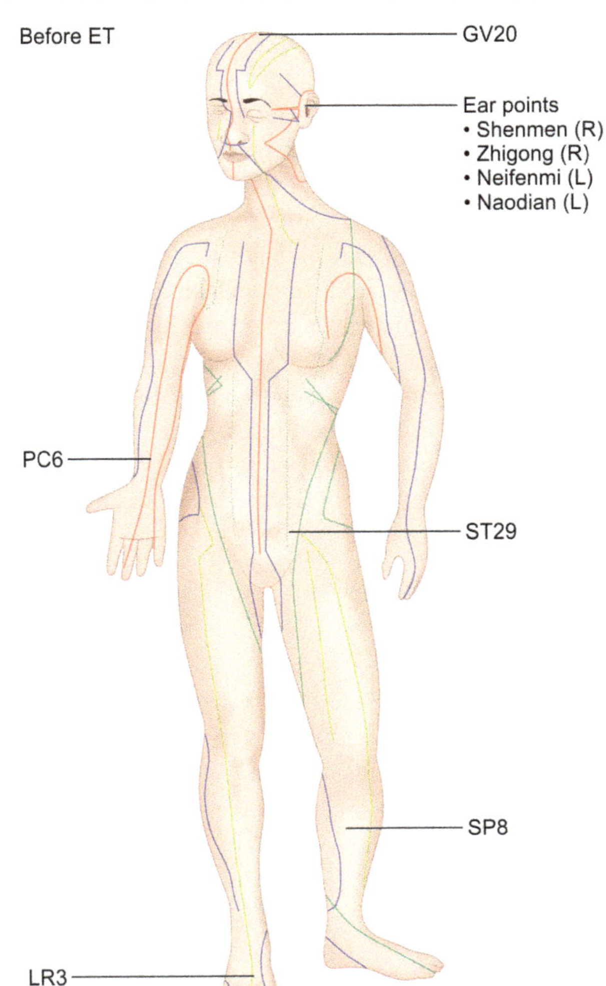

Fig. 1: Acupuncture points for fertility.
(ET: embryo transfer)
Source: Acupuncture Moxibustion. (2019). Acupuncture Moxibustion: Traditional East Asian Therapies. [online] Available from www.acupuncturemoxibustion.com. [Last accessed March, 2020].

quality of the evidence across CAM methods was poor because of improper research designs. There is a need for RCTs to determine the effectiveness of CAM in relation to fertility treatment.[96]

Surgery as an Adjuvant to Optimize In Vitro Fertilization Outcome

Routine Hysteroscopy

There is no role in routine hysteroscopy before IVF. It is required in presence of an:

- Abnormal hysterosalpingography (HSG)
- History or symptoms suggestive of endometrial or uterine pathology.

Initial studies showed benefit from pre-IVF hysteroscopy in absence of intrauterine pathology by increasing the chance of pregnancy and the number needed to treat was

6 [pooled relative risk (RR) = 1.75; 95% CI: 1.51–2.03; P < 0.00001].[97,98]

But the InSIGHT (Intervention Nurses Start Infants Growing on Healthy Trajectories) and TROPHY trials did not show any benefit of routine hysteroscopy prior to first IVF or in women with RIF.[99-101] There was another systematic review and meta-analysis which concluded that from the present data available, no firm conclusions can be made of the effect of diagnostic or operative hysteroscopy on pregnancy outcomes. It was observed that hysteroscopy or no hysteroscopy prior to any (first or subsequent) IVF/ICSI attempt in infertile women without intrauterine abnormalities does not improve LBR.[101] Comparing operative hysteroscopy for intrauterine abnormalities in infertile women with already diagnosed polyps or fibroids, there was low-quality evidence that operative hysteroscopy increases pregnancy rate (RR: 2.13; 95% CI: 1.56–2.92).[102]

The **Figures 3 and 4** highlight different surgical procedures in infertility management that have evidence and those that do not have evidence.

New Technologies Used in Assisted Reproductive Technology

After 40 years of IVF treatment and research, major progress in improving stimulation protocols and fertilization procedures, optimizing embryo culture conditions, and preventing premature luteinization, however only marginal improvement has been seen in the implantation and pregnancy rates. Variability in patient characteristics and response to ART dictate the need for proven, personalized diagnostic and therapeutic approaches to optimize efficacy and safety outcomes. Different methods of selection of gametes and embryos have been used to improve the IVF outcome **(Fig. 5)**.

Of these, spindle view and intracytoplasmic morphologically selected sperm injection (IMSI) have shown no benefit. There is some evidence for the use of physiological intracytoplasmic sperm injection (PICSI).

Blastocyst Transfer

The scientific rationale for blastocyst transfer is to increase implantation rates by improving uterine and embryonic synchronicity and allowing self-selection of embryos with greater implantation potential, but greater standardization of blastocyst morphology scales is required for this.[103-105] Though the embryo-endometrial synchrony is present with blastocyst transfer, with a higher implantation and LBR, it has a higher ET cancelation rate[106,107] with fewer embryos cryopreserved.[107,108]

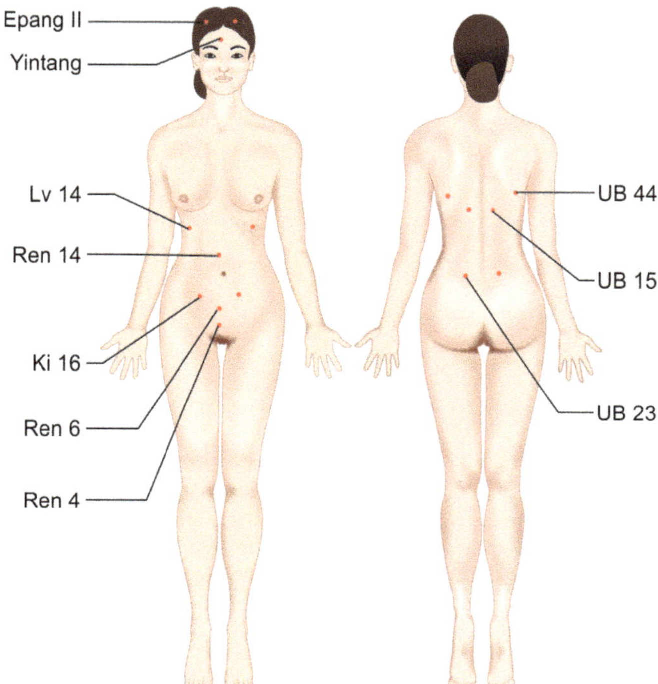

Fig. 2: Acupressure points for fertility.

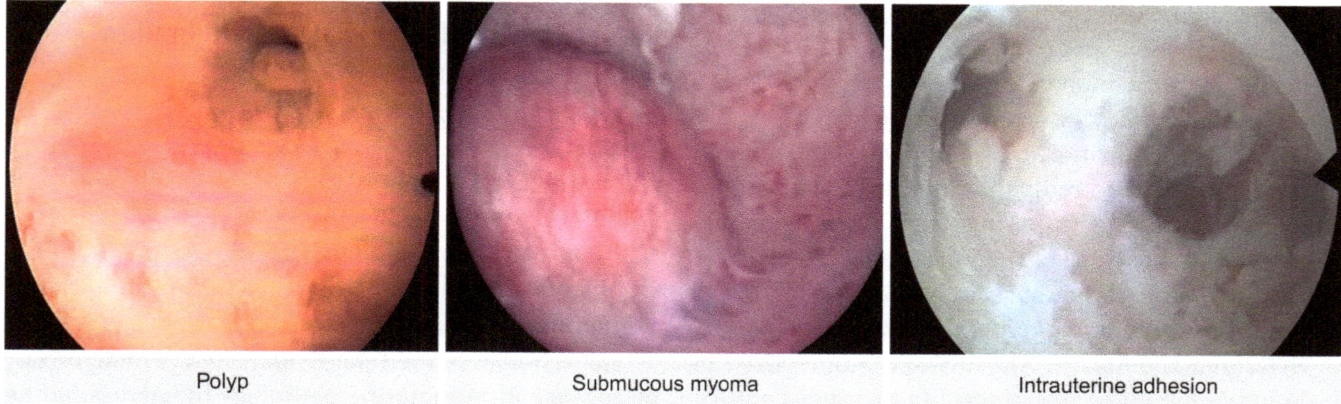

Fig. 3: Reproductive surgery indicated beyond a reasonable doubt.

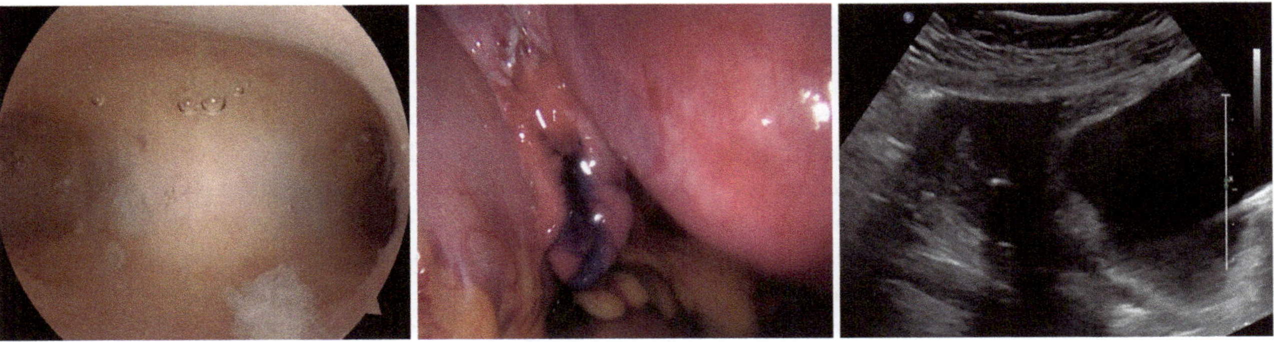

Fig. 4: Routine hysteroscopy laparoscopy and endometrial scratch.

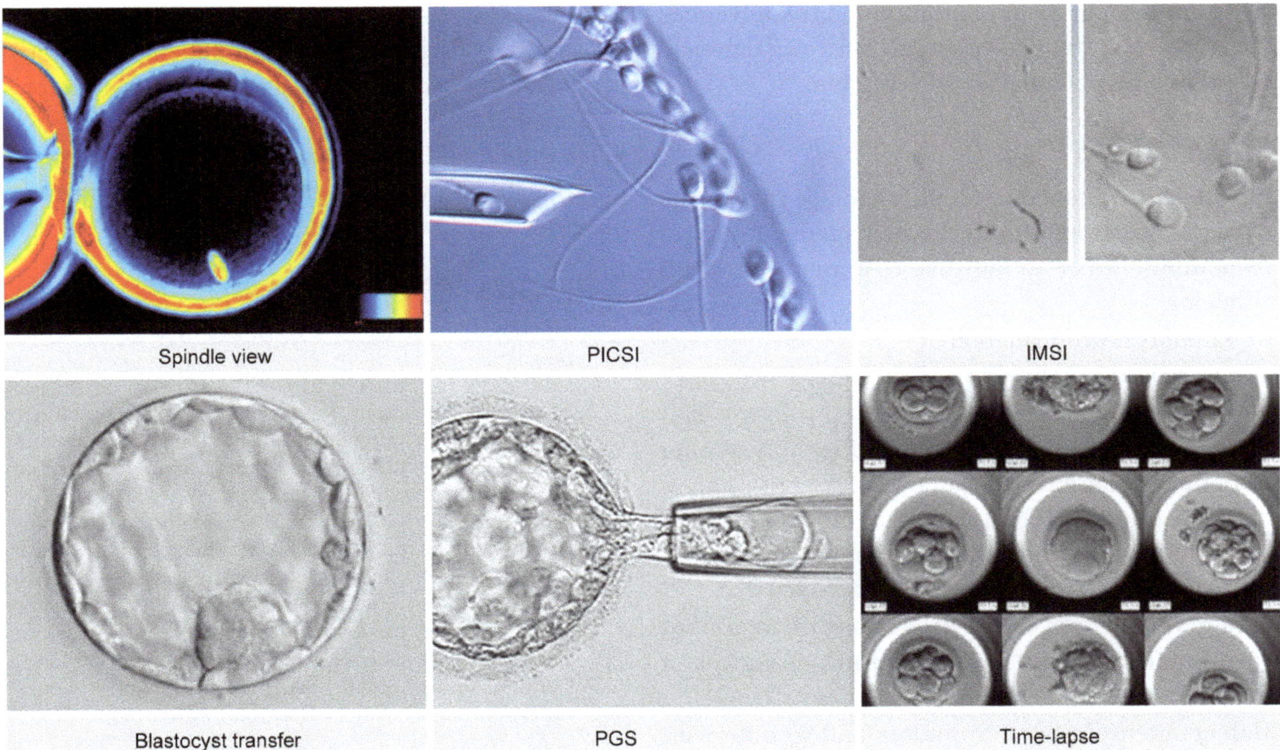

Fig. 5: Techniques used in the laboratory to improve ART outcome.
(ART: assisted reproductive technology; IMSI: intracytoplasmic morphologically selected sperm injection;
PGS: preimplantation genetic screening; PICSI: physiological intracytoplasmic sperm injection)

Time-lapse

Time-lapse is a noninvasive embryo assessment of morphokinetic parameters. Though time-lapse is a perfect tool for studying and understanding early embryo cleavages as it gives detailed information with flexibility in workflow having controlled incubation conditions and being precise, it has not yet been validated in large studies. Embryos cultured in constant and uninterrupted conditions[109] with detection of irregularities in cell cleavages which can then be deselected for ET enhancing clinical reproductive outcome.[110]

There is insufficient good-quality evidence of differences in live birth or ongoing pregnancy, miscarriage and stillbirth, or clinical pregnancy to choose between time-lapse, with or without embryo selection software, and conventional incubation.[111] Moreover, embryo culture and light exposure safety need to be evaluated and processing abundant imaging data in real-time is a challenge and is not done in most laboratories. It is also a poor predictor of IVF outcome as too many confounding factors influence the dynamics of embryo development.

Embryo Biopsy + Preimplantation Genetic Testing for Aneuploidy

Preimplantation genetic testing for aneuploidy (PGT-A) may be done to increase clinical outcomes, decrease loss rates, and decrease transfer order in IVF by transfer of euploid embryos. One must remember that PGT-A does not improve embryo quality or increase LBR. Fluorescence in situ hybridization (FISH) and day 3 biopsy have a negative impact on development and outcome of IVF with no increase in chances of having a baby.[112] The value of PGT-A as a universal screening test for all IVF patients has yet to be determined. The chances of false-positive testing, embryonic damage, and loss of euploid embryos are high, especially due to mosaicism. Other important considerations about PGT-A that must be addressed by further research include cost-effectiveness; the role and effect of cryopreservation, time to pregnancy, utility in specific subgroups (such as recurrent loss, prior implantation failure, advanced maternal age, etc.); cumulative success rates over time; and total reproductive potential per intervention.[113]

KEY MESSAGES

- Insufficient evidence to identify the use of any one particular intervention in the management of poor responders in IVF to improve treatment outcomes either for:
  - Pituitary downregulation
  - Ovarian stimulation
  - Adjuvant therapy.
- There is a need to identify those subgroups of poor responders that have theca cell failure but retain a relatively preserved GC function, as modulating their intrafollicular androgen environment by exogenous androgens may improve their ovarian response.
- Patients for whom other modalities of treatment have failed may consider the option of androgen administration.
- Management of poor responders and women with low ovarian reserve still represents a challenge for the clinician.
- Use of adjuvants in PCOS is empirical, though recent publications have shown metformin to increase pregnancy rate in gonadotropin cycles.
- Adjuvant therapy may be beneficial in preventing or reducing the severity of OHSS.
- Current evidence for adjuvants in routine IVF is still weak.
- At present, however, there is insufficient evidence to recommend the routine use of blastocyst biopsy with aneuploidy testing in all infertile patients.
- When unproven therapeutic approaches are prescribed, patients should be made aware of the lack of evidence for clinical benefits and the potential of treatment.
- Currently, little good-quality evidence to support the use of specific ART-related laboratory procedures—ICSI for all, blastocyst transfer, assisted hatching, time-lapse imaging, and freeze all.
- Evaluating the failed IVF cycle often provides useful prognostic information.
- Good medical practice dictates that the physician keeps the best interest of their patients in mind and counsel patients appropriately about the best evidence available and potential adverse effects of the treatments prescribed.
- Adaptation and personalization of fertility therapy may help to optimize efficacy and safety outcomes for individual.
- Prognostic modeling and personalized management strategies based on individual patient characteristics may prove to represent real progress toward improved treatment.
- Greater quality control and standardization of clinical and laboratory evaluations optimize ART practice and improves individual patient outcomes.

REFERENCES

1. Macklon NS, Geraedts JP, Fauser BC. Conception to ongoing pregnancy: the 'black box' of early pregnancy loss. Hum Reprod Update. 2002;8:333-43.
2. Lanzone A, Di Simone N, Castellani R, et al. Human growth hormone enhances progesterone production by human luteal cells in vitro: evidence of a synergistic effect with human chorionic gonadotropin. Fertil Steril. 1992;57:92-6.
3. Harper K, Proctor M, Hughes E. Growth hormone for in vitro fertilization. Cochrane Database Syst Rev. 2003;3:CD000099.
4. Kolibianakis EM, Venetis CA, Diedrich K, et al. Addition of growth hormone to gonadotrophins in ovarian stimulation of poor responders treated by in-vitro fertilization: a systematic review and meta-analysis. Hum Reprod Update. 2009;15:613-22.
5. Duffy JM, Ahmad G, Mohiyiddeen L, et al. Growth hormone for in vitro fertilization. Cochrane Database Syst Rev. 2010;1:CD000099.
6. Li XL, Wang L, Lv F, et al. The influence of different growth hormone addition protocols to poor ovarian responders on clinical outcomes in controlled ovary stimulation cycles: a systematic review and meta-analysis. Medicine (Baltimore). 2017;96:e6443.
7. Bayoumi YA, Dakhly DR, Bassiouny YA, et al. Addition of growth hormone to the microflare stimulation protocol among women with poor ovarian response. Int J Gynaecol Obstet. 2015;131:305-8.
8. Hart RJ, Rombauts L, Norman RJ. Growth hormone in IVF cycles: any hope? Curr Opin Obstet Gynecol. 2017;29:119-25.
9. Yu X, Ruan J, He LP, et al. Efficacy of growth hormone supplementation with gonadotrophins in vitro fertilization for poor ovarian responders: an updated meta-analysis. Int J Clin Exp Med. 2015;8:4954-67.
10. Norman RJ, Alvino H, Hull LM, et al. Human growth hormone for poor responders: a randomized placebo-controlled trial provides no evidence for improved live birth rate. Reprod Biomed Online. 2019;38:908-15.
11. Doldi N, Bassan M, Bonzi V, et al. Effects of growth hormone and growth hormone-releasing hormone on steroid synthesis in cultured human luteinizing granulosa cells. Gynecol Endocrinol. 1996;10:101-8.

12. Howles CM, Loumaye E, Germond M, et al. Does growth hormone-releasing factor assist follicular development in poor responder patients undergoing ovarian stimulation for in-vitro fertilization? Hum Reprod. 1999;14:1939-43.

13. Delitala G, Tomasi P, Virdis R. Neuroendocrine regulation of human growth hormone secretion. Diagnostic and clinical applications. J Endocrinol Invest. 1988;11:441-62.

14. Kim CH, Chae HD, Chang YS. Pyridostigmine cotreatment for controlled ovarian hyperstimulation in low responders undergoing in vitro fertilization-embryo transfer. Fertil Steril. 1999;71:652-7.

15. Chung-Hoon K, Hee-Dong C, Yoon-Seok C. Pyridostigmine cotreatment for controlled ovarian hyperstimulation in low responders undergoing in vitro fertilization ± embryo transfer. Fertil Steril. 1999;71:652-7.

16. Harlow CR, Hillier SG, Hodges JK. Androgen modulation of follicle-stimulating hormone-induced granulosa cell steroidogenesis in the primate ovary. Endocrinology. 1986;119:1403-5.

17. Hillier SG, De Zwart FA. Evidence that granulosa cell aromatase induction/activation by follicle-stimulating hormone is an androgen receptor-regulated process in-vitro. Endocrinology. 1981;109:1303-5.

18. Weil S, Vendola K, Zhou J, et al. Androgen and follicle-stimulating hormone interactions in primate ovarian follicle development. J Clin Endocrinol Metab. 1999;84:2951-6.

19. Vendola KA, Zhou J, Adesanya OO, et al. Androgens stimulate early stages of follicular growth in the primate ovary. J Clin Invest. 1998;101:2622-9.

20. Casson PR, Lindsay MS, Pisarska MD, et al. Dehydroepiandrosterone supplementation augments ovarian stimulation in poor responders: a case series. Hum Reprod. 2000;10:2129-32.

21. Balasch J, Fabregues F, Penarrubia J, et al. Pretreatment with transdermal testosterone may improve ovarian response to gonadotrophins in poor-responder IVF patients with normal basal concentrations of FSH. Hum Reprod. 2006;7:1884-93.

22. Bosdou JK, Venetis CA, Kolibianakis EM, et al. The use of androgens or androgen-modulating agents in poor responders undergoing in vitro fertilization: a systematic review and meta-analysis. Hum Reprod Update. 2012;18:127-45.

23. Bosdou JK, Venetis CA, Dafopoulos K, et al. Transdermal testosterone pretreatment in poor responders undergoing ICSI: a randomized clinical trial. Hum Reprod. 2016;31:977-85.

24. Hillier SG, Whitelaw PF, Smyth CD. Follicular oestrogen synthesis: The 'two-cell, two-gonadotrophin' model revisited. Mol Cell Endocrinol. 1994;100:51-4.

25. Barad D, Brill H, Gleicher N. Update on the use of dehydroepiandrosterone supplementation among women with diminished ovarian function. J Assist Reprod Genet. 2007;24:629-34.

26. Hyman EJ, Margalioth EJ, Rabinowitz R, et al. Dehydro-epiandrosterone (DHEA) supplementation for poor responders-how does it work? Fertil Steril. 2010;94:S86.

27. Mamas L, Mamas E. Premature ovarian failure and dehydroepiandrosterone. Fertil Steril. 2009;91:644-6.

28. Sönmezer M, Cil AP, Oktay K. Ongoing pregnancies from early retrieval of prematurely developing antral follicles after DHEA supplementation. Reprod Biomed Online. 2009;19:816-9.

29. Wiser A, Gonen O, Ghetler Y, et al. Addition of dehydroepiandrosterone (DHEA) for poor-responder patients before and during IVF treatment improves the pregnancy rate: a randomized prospective study. Hum Reprod. 2010;25:2496-500.

30. Narkwichean A, Maalouf W, Campbell BK, et al. Efficacy of dehydroepiandrosterone to improve ovarian response in women with diminished ovarian reserve: a meta-analysis. Reprod Biol Endocrinol. 2013;11:44.

31. Ubaldi F, Vaiarelli A, D'Anna R, et al. Management of poor responders in IVF: is there anything new? Biomed Res Int. 2014;2014:352098.

32. Xu B, Li Z, Yue J, et al. Effect of dehydroepiandrosterone administration in patients with poor ovarian response according to the Bologna criteria. PLoS One. 2014;9:e99858.

33. Gleicher N, Weghofer A, Barad DH. Dehydroepiandrosterone (DHEA) reduces embryo aneuploidy: direct evidence from preimplantation genetic screening (PGS). Reprod Biol Endocrinol. 2010;8:140.

34. Gleicher N, Weghofer A, Barad DH. Discordances between follicle stimulating hormone (FSH) and anti-Müllerian hormone (AMH) in female infertility. Reprod Biol Endocrinol. 2010;8:64.

35. Borman E, Check JH, Williams JM, et al. No evidence to support the concept that low serum dehydroepiandrosterone (DHEA) sulphate (S) levels are associated with less oocyte production or lower pregnancy rates. Clin Exp Obstet Gynecol. 2012;39:429-31.

36. Motta EL, Rossi LM, Fernandes TR, et al. The use of DHEA in poor responders does not improve IVF outcomes: insights of a pilot study. Fertil Steril. 2006;86:S428.

37. Yakin K, Urman B. DHEA as a miracle drug in the treatment of poor responders; hype or hope? Hum Reprod. 2011;26:1941-4.

38. Sönmezer M, Ozmen B, Cil AP, et al. Dehydroepiandrosterone supplementation improves ovarian response and cycle outcome in poor responders. Reprod Biomed Online. 2009;19:508-13.

39. Sciard C, Berthiller J, Brosse A, et al. Preliminary results of DHEA in poor responders in IVF. Open J Obstet Gynecol. 2016;6:396-403.

40. Zhang M, Niu W, Wang Y, et al. Dehydroepiandrosterone treatment in women with poor ovarian response undergoing IVF or ICSI: a systematic review and meta-analysis. J Assist Reprod Genet. 2016;33:981-91.

41. Szymusik I, Marianowski P, Zygula A, et al. Poor responders in IVF—is there any evidence-based treatment for them? Neuro Endocrinol Lett. 2015;36:209-13.

42. González-Comadran M, Durán M, Solà I, et al. Effects of transdermal testosterone in poor responders undergoing IVF: systematic review and meta-analysis. Reprod Biomed Online. 2012;25:450-9.

43. Polyzos NP, Davis SR, Drakopoulos P, et al. Testosterone for poor ovarian responders: lessons from ovarian physiology. Reprod Sci. 2016;25:980-2.

44. Gelbaya TA, Kyrgiou M, Li TC, et al. Low-dose aspirin for in vitro fertilization: a systematic review and meta-analysis. Hum Reprod Update. 2007;13:357-64.

45. Lok IH, Yip SK, Cheung LP, et al. Adjuvant low-dose aspirin therapy in poor responders undergoing in vitro fertilization: a prospective, randomized, double-blind, placebo-controlled trial. Fertil Steril. 2004;81:556-61.

46. Weckstein LN, Jacobson A, Galen D, et al. Low-dose aspirin for oocyte donation recipients with a thin endometrium: prospective, randomized study. Fertil Steril. 1997;68:927-30.

47. Khairy M, Banerjee K, El-Toukhy T, et al. Aspirin in women undergoing in vitro fertilization treatment: a systematic review and meta-analysis. Fertil Steril. 2007;88:822-31.

48. Revelli A, Dolfin E, Gennarelli G, et al. Low-dose acetylsalicylic acid plus prednisolone as an adjuvant treatment in IVF: a prospective, randomized study. Fertil Steril. 2008;90:1685-91.

49. Ruopp MD, Collins TC, Whitcomb BW, et al. Evidence of absence or absence of evidence? A reanalysis of the effects of low-dose aspirin in in vitro fertilization. Fertil Steril. 2008;90:71-6.

50. Battaglia C, Regnani G, Marsella T, et al. Adjuvant L-arginine treatment in controlled ovarian hyperstimulation: a double-blind, randomized study. Hum Reprod. 2002;17:659-65.

51. Tartagni M, Cicinelli E, De Pergola G, et al. Effects of pretreatment with estrogens on ovarian stimulation with gonadotropins in

women with premature ovarian failure: a randomized, placebo-controlled trial. Fertil Steril. 2007;87:858-61.

52. Takasaki A, Ohba T, Okamura Y, et al. Clinical use of colony-stimulating factor-1 in ovulation induction for poor responders. Fertil Steril. 2008;90:2287-90.

53. Ebrahimi M, Akbari-Asbagh F, Ghalandar-Attar M. Letrozole + GnRH antagonist stimulation protocol in poor ovarian responders undergoing intracytoplasmic sperm injection cycles: An RCT. Int J Reprod Biomed (Yazd). 2017;15:101-8.

54. Fouda UM, Sayed AM. Extended high dose letrozole regimen versus short low dose letrozole regimen as an adjuvant to gonadotropin releasing hormone antagonist protocol in poor responders undergoing IVF-ET. Gynecol Endocrinol. 2011;27:1018-22.

55. Yarali H, Esinler İ, Polat M, et al. Antagonist/letrozole protocol in poor ovarian responders for intracytoplasmic sperm injection: a comparative study with the microdose flare-up protocol. Fertil Steril. 2009;92:231-5.

56. Begum MR, Ehsan M, Begum MS, et al. Beneficial effects of addition of glucocorticoid during induction of ovulation by letrozole in polycystic ovarian syndrome. J South Asian Fed Obstet Gynaecol. 2012;4:85-9.

57. Macklon N, Fauser BC. Medical approaches to ovarian stimulation for infertility. Reprod Endocrinol. 2009;2:689-724.

58. Parsanezhad M, Alborzi S, Motazedian S, et al. Use of dexamethasone and clomiphene citrate in the treatment of clomiphene citrate-resistant patients with polycystic ovary syndrome and normal dehydroepiandrosterone sulfate levels: a prospective, double-blind, placebo-controlled trial. Fertil Steril. 2002;78:1001-4.

59. Tso LO, Costello MF, Albuquerque LE, et al. Metformin treatment before and during IVF or ICSI in women with polycystic ovary syndrome. Cochrane Database Syst Rev. 2014;11:CD006105.

60. Usadi RS, Merriam KS. On-label and off-label drug use in the treatment of female infertility. Fertil Steril. 2015;103:583-94.

61. Bordewijk EM, Nahuis M, Costello MF, et al. Metformin during ovulation induction with gonadotrophins followed by timed intercourse or intrauterine insemination for subfertility associated with polycystic ovary syndrome. Cochrane Database Syst Rev. 2017;1:CD009090.

62. Morley LC, Tang T, Yasmin E, et al. Insulin-sensitising drugs (metformin, rosiglitazone, pioglitazone, D-chiro-inositol) for women with polycystic ovary syndrome, oligo amenorrhoea and subfertility. Cochrane Database Syst Rev. 2017;11:CD003053.

63. Baillargeon JP, Diamanti-Kandarakis E, Ostlund RE, et al. Altered D-chiro-inositol urinary clearance in women with polycystic ovary syndrome. Diabetes Care. 2006;29:300-5.

64. Unfer V, Carlomagno G, Dante G, et al. Effects of myo-inositol in women with PCOS: a systematic review of randomized controlled trials. Gynecol Endocrinol. 2012;28:509-15.

65. Regidor PA, Schindler AE. Myoinositol as a safe and alternative approach in the treatment of infertile PCOS women: a German observational study. Int J Endocrinol. 2016;2016:9537632.

66. Garg D, Tal R. Inositol treatment and ART outcomes in women with PCOS. Int J Endocrinol. 2016;2016:1979654.

67. Salehpour S, Sene AA, Saharkhiz N, et al. N-acetylcysteine as an adjuvant to clomiphene citrate for successful induction of ovulation in infertile patients with polycystic ovary syndrome. J Obstet Gynaecol Res. 2012;38:1182-6.

68. Maged AM, Elsawah H, Abdelhafez A, et al. The adjuvant effect of metformin and N-acetylcysteine to clomiphene citrate in induction of ovulation in patients with polycystic ovary syndrome. Gynecol Endocrinol. 2015;31:635-8.

69. Basheer M, Rai S, Hsu TC. Melatonin vs. phytomelatonin: therapeutic uses with special reference to polycystic ovarian syndrome (PCOS). Cogent Biol. 2016;2:1136257.

70. Fernando S, Rombauts L. Melatonin: shedding light on infertility?—a review of the recent literature. J Ovarian Res. 2014;7:98.

71. Seko LM, Moroni RM, Leitao VM, et al. Melatonin supplementation during controlled ovarian stimulation for women undergoing assisted reproductive technology: systematic review and meta-analysis of randomized controlled trials. Fertil Steril. 2014;101:154-61.e4.

72. Irani M, Merhi Z. Role of vitamin D in ovarian physiology and its implication in reproduction: a systemic review. Fertil Steril. 2014;102:460-8.e3.

73. Deshpande H. Practical Management of Ovulation Induction. New Delhi: Jaypee Brothers Medical Publishers (P) Pvt. Ltd.; 2016.

74. El-Refaeey A, Selem A, Badawy A. Combined coenzyme Q10 and clomiphene citrate for ovulation induction in clomiphene-citrate-resistant polycystic ovary syndrome. Reprod Biomed Online. 2014;29:119-24.

75. Stephenson MD, Fluker MR. Treatment of repeated unexplained in vitro fertilization failure with intravenous immunoglobulin: a randomized, placebo-controlled Canadian trial. Fertil Steril. 2000;74:1108-13.

76. Clark DA, Coulam CB, Stricker RB. Is intravenous immunoglobulins (IVIG) efficacious in early pregnancy failure? A critical review and meta-analysis for patients who fail in vitro fertilization and embryo transfer (IVF). J Assist Reprod Genet. 2006;23:1-3.

77. Sherer Y, Levy Y, Langevitz P, et al. Adverse effects of intravenous immunoglobulin therapy in 56 patients with autoimmune diseases. Pharmacology. 2001;62:133-7.

78. Boomsma CM, Keay SD, Macklon NS. Peri-implantation glucocorticoid administration for assisted reproductive technology cycles. Cochrane Database Syst Rev. 2012;6:CD005996.

79. Check JH, Graziano V, Lee G, et al. Neither sildenafil nor vaginal estradiol improves endometrial thickness in women with thin endometrial after taking oral estradiol in graduating dosages. Clin Exp Obstet Gynecol. 2004;31:99-102.

80. Kutteh WH. Antiphospholipid antibody-associated recurrent pregnancy loss: treatment with heparin and low-dose aspirin is superior to low-dose aspirin alone. Am J Obstet Gynecol. 1996;174:1584-9.

81. Tulppala M, Marttunen M, Söderstrom-Anttila V, et al. Low-dose aspirin in prevention of miscarriage in women with unexplained or autoimmune related recurrent miscarriage: effect on prostacyclin and thromboxane A2 production. Hum Reprod. 1997;12:1567-72.

82. Stern C, Chamley L, Hale L, et al. Antibodies to β2 glycoprotein I are associated with in vitro fertilization implantation failure as well as recurrent miscarriage: results of a prevalence study. Fertil Steril. 1998;70:938-44.

83. Urman B, Ata B, Yakin K, et al. Luteal phase empirical low molecular weight heparin administration in patients with failed ICSI embryo transfer cycles: a randomized open-labeled pilot trial. Hum Reprod. 2009;24:1640-7.

84. Akhtar MA, Eljabu H, Hopkisson J, et al. Aspirin and heparin as adjuvants during IVF do not improve live birth rates in unexplained implantation failure. Reprod Biomed Online. 2013;26:586-94.

85. Noci I, Milanini MN, Ruggiero M, et al. Effect of dalteparin sodium administration on IVF outcome in non-thrombophilic young women: a pilot study. Reprod Biomed Online. 2011;22:615-20.

86. Stern C, Chamley L, Norris H, et al. A randomized, double-blind, placebo-controlled trial of heparin and aspirin for women with in vitro fertilization implantation failure and antiphospholipid or antinuclear antibodies. Fertil Steril. 2003;80:376-83.

87. Sher G, Feinman M, Zouves C, et al. High fecundity rates following in-vitro fertilization and embryo transfer in antiphospholipid antibody seropositive women treated with heparin and aspirin. Hum Reprod. 1994;9:2278-83.

88. Simon A, Laufer N. Assessment and treatment of repeated implantation failure (RIF). J Assist Reprod Genet. 2012;29: 1227-39.

89. Hamdi K, Danaii S, Farzadi L, et al. The role of heparin in embryo implantation in women with recurrent implantation failure in the cycles of assisted reproductive techniques (without history of thrombophilia). J Family Reprod Health. 2015;9:59-64.

90. Luddi A, Capaldo A, Focarelli R, et al. Antioxidants reduce oxidative stress in follicular fluid of aged women undergoing IVF. Reprod Biol Endocrinol. 2016;14:57.

91. Wang S, He G, Chen M, et al. The role of antioxidant enzymes in the ovaries. Oxid Med Cell Long. 2017;2017:4371714.

92. Cheong YC, Ng EH, Ledger WL. Acupuncture and assisted conception. Cochrane Database Syst Rev. 2008;4:CD006920.

93. Kovárová P, Smith CA, Turnbull DA. An exploratory study of the effect of acupuncture on self-efficacy for women seeking fertility support. Explore (NY). 2010;6:330-4.

94. Cheong KB, Zhang JP, Huang Y, et al. The effectiveness of acupuncture in prevention and treatment of postoperative nausea and vomiting—a systematic review and meta-analysis. PLoS One. 2013;8:e82474.

95. Okhowat J, Murtinger M, Schuff M, et al. Massage therapy improves in vitro fertilization outcome in patients undergoing blastocyst transfer in a cryo-cyde. Alternative Therapies in Health & Medicine. 2015;21(2).

96. Miner SA, Robins S, Zhu YJ, et al. Evidence for the use of complementary and alternative medicines during fertility treatment: a scoping review. BMC Complement Altern Med. 2018;18:158.

97. El-Toukhy T, Sunkara SK, Coomarasamy A, et al. Outpatient hysteroscopy and subsequent IVF cycle outcome: a systematic review and meta-analysis. Reprod Biomed Online. 2008;16:712-9.

98. Bosteels J, Weyers S, Puttemans P, et al. The effectiveness of hysteroscopy in improving pregnancy rates in subfertile women without other gynaecological symptoms: a systematic review. Hum Reprod Update. 2010;16:1-11.

99. Smit JG, Kasius JC, Eijkemans MJ, et al. The inSIGHT study: costs and effects of routine hysteroscopy prior to a first IVF treatment cycle. A randomised controlled trial. BMC Womens Health. 2012;12:22.

100. Smit JG, Kasius JC, Eijkemans MJ, et al. Hysteroscopy before in-vitro fertilisation (inSIGHT): a multicentre, randomised controlled trial. Lancet. 2016;387:2622-9.

101. El-Toukhy T, Campo R, Khalaf Y, et al. Hysteroscopy in recurrent in-vitro fertilisation failure (TROPHY): a multicentre, randomised controlled trial. Lancet. 2016;387:2614-21.

102. Di Spiezio Sardo A, Di Carlo C, Minozzi S, et al. Efficacy of hysteroscopy in improving reproductive outcomes of infertile couples: a systematic review and meta-analysis. Hum Reprod Update. 2016;22:479-96.

103. Wilson M, Hartke K, Kiehl M, et al. Integration of blastocyst transfer for all patients. Fertil Steril. 2002;77:693-6.

104. Blake DA, Farquhar CM, Johnson N, et al. Cleavage stage versus blastocyst stage embryo transfer in assisted conception. Cochrane Database Syst Rev. 2007;17:CD002118.

105. Montag M, Toth B, Strowitzki T. New approaches to embryo selection. Reprod Biomed Online. 2013;27:539-46.

106. Marek D, Langley M, Gardner DK, et al. Introduction of blastocyst culture and transfer for all patients in an in vitro fertilization program. Fertil Steril. 1999;72:1035-40.

107. Papanikolaou EG, D'haeseleer E, Verheyen G, et al. Live birth rate is significantly higher after blastocyst transfer than after cleavage-stage embryo transfer when at least four embryos are available on day 3 of embryo culture. A randomized prospective study. Hum Reprod. 2005;20:3198-203.

108. Tsirigotis M. Blastocyst stage transfer: pitfalls and benefits. Too soon to abandon current practice? Hum Reprod. 2008;13:3285-9.

109. Ciray HN, Campbell A, Agerholm IE, et al. Proposed guidelines on the nomenclature and annotation of dynamic human embryo monitoring by a time-lapse user group. Hum Reprod. 2014;29:2650-60.

110. Hojnik N, Vlaisavljević V, Kovačič B. Morphokinetic characteristics and developmental potential of in vitro cultured embryos from natural cycles in patients with poor ovarian response. Biomed Res Int. 2016;2016:4286528.

111. Armstrong S, Bhide P, Jordan V, et al. Time-lapse systems for embryo incubation and assessment in assisted reproduction. Cochrane Database Syst Rev. 2018;5:CD011320.

112. Twisk M, Mastenbroek S, Hoek A, et al. No beneficial effect of preimplantation genetic screening in women of advanced maternal age with a high risk for embryonic aneuploidy. Hum Reprod. 2008;23:2813-7.

113. Penzias A, Bendikson K, Butts S, et al. The use of preimplantation genetic testing for aneuploidy (PGT-A): a committee opinion. Fertil Steril. 2018;109:429-36.

Current Controversies and Consensus for Adjuvants in Polycystic Ovary Syndrome

Sujata Kar

INTRODUCTION

Polycystic ovary syndrome (PCOS) is the most common multiorgan endocrinopathy affecting women of reproductive age group. This reproductive and cardiometabolic syndrome greatly increasing a woman's lifetime risk of infertility, menstrual abnormalities, type II diabetes mellitus, and cardiovascular diseases. A cure is being highly sought after by researchers. But in the absence of a known pathophysiologic mechanism, this appears to be elusive. Currently, various investigational therapies, targeting many symptoms of PCOS, are being tried. Present article attempts to enumerate such therapies and explore their current status.

INSULIN-SENSITIZING AGENTS

Polycystic ovary syndrome women, both obese and normal weight, have a very high prevalence of insulin resistance and hyperinsulinemia. Thus, the rationale to use insulin-sensitizing agents in PCOS women is very strong. Biguanides and thiazolidinediones have been used extensively and large body of data exists on this subject. Some other novel agents which likely affect insulin resistance and metabolic profile of the PCOS woman have been discussed in this article.

SOMATOSTATIN ANALOGS

Somatostatin is an endogenous hypothalamic peptide with 14 amino acids and a short half-life. It inhibits pancreatic insulin release, pituitary growth hormone secretion, and also luteinizing hormone (LH) release in response of gonadotropin-releasing hormone (GnRH).[1-3] This property therefore should be useful in PCOS management. Somatostatin analog octreotide has been shown in few studies to improve pulsatile gonadotropin patterns, reduced LH, androgen and insulin-like growth factor-1 (IGF-1) levels, and improved ovulation.[4-12] Octreotide (LAR), long-acting somatostatin analog formulations, has also been tried and shown to directly influence insulin secretion.[3,13-15] Thus, this drug has potential role as insulin-sensitizing agent, improves hyperinsulinemia as well as has direct effect on the ovaries as suggested by recent discovery of somatostatin receptors at ovarian levels.[16]

INOSITOLS

"Inositol" is a group of naturally occurring carbohydrate compounds, which plays a small but significant role in "insulin" signaling. Many studies have reported defective inositol signaling as likely pathologic mechanism for insulin resistance of PCOS women. Three inositol family members have been tried in PCOS: (1) D-chiro-inositol (DCI), (2) myoinositol and (3) D-pinitol. These new molecules are thought to be having insulin-sensitizing properties, likely to improve metabolic, cardiovascular, and reproductive profiles of PCOS women. There are many studies reporting the use of inositols in reducing insulin resistance and dyslipidemias in PCOS women.[17]

In a recent paper,[18] combination of myoinositol and DCI, in a physiologic ratio of 40:1, was shown to improve metabolic profile of PCOS women. Also, in another study, this combination therapy was shown to improve oocyte, embryo quality, and pregnancy rates in PCOS women undergoing in vitro fertilization (IVF)-embryo transfer (ET).[17]

Artini et al. studied 50 overweight PCOS women before and after 12 weeks course of myoinositol 2 g with folic acid 200 mg daily. Patients were randomized to either the above combination or to only folic acid 200 mg daily.[19] They reported that after 12 weeks of myoinositol administration, plasma LH, prolactin, testosterone, insulin levels, and LH/follicle-stimulating hormone (FSH) were significantly reduced. Insulin sensitivity expressed as glucose to insulin ratio and homeostatic model assessment (HOMA) index significantly improved. Menstrual cyclicity was restored in all amenorrheic and oligomenorrheic subjects. No such improvement was seen in "folic acid only" group. A systematic review[20] published in 2011 looked into the effects of DCI on ovulation and insulin resistance in women with PCOS. All studies published on PCOS and DCI up to 2010 were included. Patients were women with PCOS receiving DCI or where the relationship between insulin resistance and DCI had been investigated. Ovulation rates and insulin resistance were the main outcome measures. They concluded that heterogeneity in study methodologies and small sample size used prohibit reliable conclusions to be drawn. More studies are needed to evaluate accurately the effects of DCI in PCOS. The inositols have potential to improved reproductive axis functioning by reducing hyperinsulinemia.

N-ACETYLCYSTEINE

N-acetylcysteine (NAC) is a pharmaceutical drug and also nutritional supplement. Acetylcysteine is the N-acetyl derivative of amino acid L-cysteine which forms antioxidant glutathione in the body. This compound is sold commonly as a dietary supplement, claiming antioxidant, and liver protecting effects. Recent studies have shown beneficial effects from the use of NAC for patients with PCOS. Oner et al. reported clinical, endocrine, and metabolic effects of metformin and NAC in PCOS women.[21] In this prospective trial, 100 women with PCOS were randomly divided to receive metformin (1,500 mg/day) or NAC (1,800 mg/day) for 24 weeks. Both treatments resulted in a significant decrease in body mass index, hirsutism score, fasting insulin, HOMA index, free testosterone, and menstrual irregularity, compared with baseline values. Also, both treatments have equal efficacy. NAC reduced both total and low-density lipoproteins whereas metformin only led to a decrease in total cholesterol.

Ritz et al.[22] studied NAC as a novel adjuvant to clomiphene citrate (CC) in CC-resistant PCOS women. 150 women diagnosed with CC-resistant PCOS, aged 18–39 years, undergoing infertility treatment were included. The women were randomized to receive either NAC (1.2 g/day) or placebo with CC (100 mg/day). Ovulation rates and pregnancy rates were reported. They concluded that NAC as an adjuvant was more effective than placebo for CC-resistant PCOS women. Nasr studied effect of NAC after ovulation drilling in CC-resistant PCOS women.

60 CC-resistant women who had undergone unilateral laparoscopic ovarian drilling were randomized to receive placebo or NAC (1.2 g/day) for 12 consecutive cycles. Ovulation rate, pregnancy rate, and live birth rate were all significantly higher in the NAC group.[23] Thus, there is now a large body of evidence to support the use of NAC in women with PCOS. It is likely to help in the following conditions: to improve insulin sensitivity, to restore fertility, and also to tackle homocysteine levels. It has been shown that many women with PCOS have high homocysteine levels.[22] Elevated homocysteine is associated with coronary artery disease, myocardial infarction, chronic fatigue, fibromyalgia, and cervical cancer. A 2009 study showed that people taking NAC for 2 months had a significant decrease in homocysteine levels.[24]

25-HYDROXYVITAMIN D

Vitamin D deficiency has been shown to be prevalent in PCOS women.[25] About 65–85% of women with PCOS have serum concentration of 25-hydroxyvitamin D (25-OH Vitamin D) < 20 ng/mL. Some observational studies have shown that lower 25-OH Vitamin D levels are associated with insulin resistance, ovulatory and menstrual irregularities, hirsutism, hyperandrogenism, obesity, and elevated cardiovascular risk factors.

Pal et al.[26] studied 12 overweight, vitamin D-deficient, PCOS women. Blood pressure, plasma glucose, total testosterone, serum sex hormone-binding globulin, and 2-hour oral glucose tolerance test were assessed at baseline and after 3 months therapy with vitamin D and elemental calcium. Their results showed improved androgen and blood pressure profile. However, glucose and insulin resistance parameters remained unchanged.

Wehr et al. studied 57 PCOS women, who received 20,000 IU cholecalciferol weekly for 24 weeks. Anthropometric measures, oral glucose tolerance test, and blood analyses of endocrine parameters were performed at baseline after 12 weeks and also after 24 weeks.

Their results showed improved glucose metabolism and menstrual frequency in these women, but no changes in androgens.[27] Thus, vitamin D deficiency may play a role in exacerbating PCOS and there may be a role for vitamin D supplementation in the management of this syndrome, but current evidence is limited. Additional randomized controlled trials are needed to confirm place of vitamin D in management of PCOS.[25]

MAGNESIUM

There are some reports linking hypomagnesemia with PCOS. Whether serum magnesium concentrations correlate with insulin resistance and hypertension, dyslipidemias of PCOS women are currently unknown. Kauffman et al. in 100 PCOS women could not find any correlation between PCOS and non-PCOS women in their magnesium levels.[28] Sharifi et al.[29] too could not find any evidence to show that magnesium deficiency is associated with insulin resistance of PCOS. However, a very recent study reported in 2013, Chakraborty et al. studied 132 PCOS women for multiple trace elements including copper, magnesium, zinc, manganese, chromium, and calcium. Further, they also divided PCOS women into insulin resistant and noninsulin resistant. They found highly significant correlation between low serum calcium and magnesium levels with insulin resistance in PCOS women.[30]

LIPOIC ACID

Alpha-lipoic acid is a potent antioxidant. We know that oxidative stress is a likely mechanism leading to insulin resistance in PCOS women. Controlled-release alpha lipoic acid (CRLA) has been reported to improve glucose control in type 2 diabetic patients.[31] Masharani et al. have reported the effects of CRLA on the features of PCOS women. Six lean, nondiabetic PCOS women were given CRLA 600 mg twice daily for 16 weeks. Insulin sensitivity was measured by euglycemic-hyperinsulinemic clamp; plasma lipids and serum oxidative markers were measured. Results showed a significant improvement in insulin sensitivity and a lowering of triglyceride levels. This was however not associated with increase in plasma antioxidant capacity.[32] They concluded that CRLA has positive effects on PCOS phenotype. This agent needs further studies to substantiate its likely benefits.

OMEGA-3 FATTY ACIDS

A link between PCOS and nonalcoholic fatty liver disease (NAFLD) has been demonstrated for few years now. Prevalence of NAFLD in women with PCOS may be as high as 40–55%.[33,34] NAFLD is characterized by increased hepatic storage of triglycerides and carries risk of cirrhosis. Very few published studies have tested various treatment options for NAFLD in association with PCOS. Animal studies of marine-derived omega-3 fatty acids have demonstrated beneficial effects in NAFLD.[35]

Cussons et al. published in 2009 a study that examined the effects of omega-3 fatty acids on liver fat in PCOS. 25 PCOS women were randomized to receive 4 g/day of omega-3 fatty acids or placebo for 8 weeks. They concluded that omega-3 fatty acid supplementation had a beneficial effect on liver fat content and other cardiovascular risk factors in women with PCOS, including those with hepatic steatosis.[36]

Mohammadi et al., in a double-blind randomized controlled trial conducted on 64 PCOS patients, concluded that omega-3 fatty acids had some beneficial effects on serum adiponectin levels, insulin resistance, and lipid profile in PCOS patients and may contribute to the improvement of metabolic complications in these women.[37]

REFERENCES

1. Chiodera P, Volpi R, d'Amato L, et al. Inhibition by somatostatin of LH-RH-induced LH release in normal menstruating women. Gynecol Obstet Invest. 1986;22:17-21.
2. Brazaan JC, Vale W, Burgus N, et al. Hypothalamic polypeptide that inhibits the secretion of immunoreactive pituitary growth hormone. Science. 1973;179:77-9.
3. Hsu WH, Xiang HD, Rajan AS, et al. Somatostatin inhibits insulin secretion by a G-protein-mediated decrease in Ca^{2+} entry through voltage-dependent Ca^{2+} channels in the beta-cell. J Biol Chem. 1991;266:837-43.
4. Prevelić GM, Wurzburger MI, Balint-Perić L, et al. Inhibitory effect of sandostatin on secretion of luteinizing hormone and ovarian steroids in polycystic ovary syndrome. Lancet. 1990;336:900-3.
5. Prelević GM, Wurzburger MI, Balint-Perić L, et al. Effects of the somatostatin analogue, octreotide, in polycystic ovary syndrome. Metabolism. 1992;41:76-9.
6. Prelević GM, Ginsburg J, Maletic D, et al. The effects of the somatostatin analogue octreotide on ovulatory performance in women with polycystic ovaries. Hum Reprod. 1995;10:28-32.
7. Morris RS, Carmina E, Vijod MA, et al. Alterations in the sensitivity of serum insulin-like growth factor 1 and insulin-like growth factor binding protein-3 to octreotide in polycystic ovary syndrome. Fertil Steril. 1995;63:742-6.
8. Fulghesu AM, Lanzone A, Andreani CL, et al. Effectiveness of a somatostatin analogue in lowering luteinizing hormone and insulin stimulated secretion in hyperinsulinemic women with polycystic ovary disease. Fertil Steril. 1995;64:703-8.
9. Morris RS, Karande VC, Dudkiewicz A, et al. Octreotide is not useful for clomiphene citrate resistance in patients with polycystic ovary syndrome but may reduce the likelihood of ovarian hyperstimulation syndrome. Fertil Steril. 1999;71:452-6.
10. Lidor A, Soriano D, Seidman DS, et al. Combined somatostatin analog and follicle-stimulating hormone for women with polycystic ovary syndrome resistant to conventional treatment. Gynecol Endocrinol. 1998;12:97-101.
11. Ciotta L, De Leo V, Galvani F, et al. Endocrine and metabolic effects of octreotide, a somatostatin analogue, in lean PCOS patients with either hyperinsulinemia or normoinsulinemia. Hum Reprod. 1999;14:2951-8.
12. Wenzl R, Lehner R, Schurz B, et al. Successful ovulation induction by sandostatin-therapy of polycystic ovarian disease. Acta Obstet Gynecol Scand. 1996;75:298-9.
13. Gambineri A, Patton L, De Iasio R, et al. Efficacy of octreotide-LAR in dieting women with abdominal obesity and polycystic ovary syndrome. J Clin Endocrinol Metab. 2005;90:3854-62.
14. Gillis JC, Noble S, Goa KL. Octreotide long-acting release (LAR): a review of its pharmacological properties and therapeutic use in the management of acromegaly. Drugs. 1997;53:681-99.
15. Bertoli A, Magnaterra R, Borboni P, et al. Dose-dependent effect of octreotide on insulin secretion after OGTT in obesity. Horm Res. 1998;49:17-21.
16. Strass MC, Seelig AS, Weiss JM, et al. Expression of somatostatin and its receptors in human ovary. 19th Annual Meeting of the ESHRE 2003. Fertil Steril. 2003;165:495.

17. Colazingari S, Treglia M, Najjar R, et al. The combined therapy myo-inositol plus D-chiro-inositol, rather than D-chiro-inositol, is able to improve IVF outcomes: results from a randomized controlled trial. Arch Gynecol Obstet. 2013;288:1405-11.

18. Minozzi M, Nordio M, Pajalich R. The combined therapy myo-inositol plus D-chiro-inositol, in a physiological ratio, reduces the cardiovascular risk by improving the lipid profile in PCOS patients. Eur Rev Med Pharmacol Sci. 2013;17:537-40.

19. Artini PG, Di Berardino OM, Papini F, et al. Endocrine and clinical effects of myo-inositol administration in polycystic ovary syndrome: a randomized study. Gynecol Endocrinol. 2013;29:375-9.

20. Galazis N, Galazi M, Atiomo W. D-chiro-inositol and its significance in polycystic ovary syndrome: a systematic review. Gynecol Endocrinol. 2011;27:256-62.

21. Oner G, Muderris II. Clinical, endocrine and metabolic effects of metformin vs N-acetyl-cysteine in women with polycystic ovary syndrome. Eur J Obstet Gynecol Reprod Biol. 2011;159:127-31.

22. Rizk AY, Ritz et al MA, Al-Inany HG. N-acetyl-cysteine is a novel adjuvant to clomiphene citrate in clomiphene citrate-resistant patients with polycystic ovary syndrome. Fertil Steril. 2005;83:367-70.

23. Nasr A. Effect of N-acetyl-cysteine after ovarian drilling in clomiphene citrate-resistant PCOS women: a pilot study. Reprod Biomed Online. 2010;20:403-9.

24. Rymarz A, Durlik M, Rydzewski A. Intravenous administration of N-acetylcysteine reduces plasma total homocysteine levels in renal transplant recipients. Transplant. 2009;14:5-9.

25. Thomson RL, Spedding S, Buckley JD. Vitamin D in the aetiology and management of polycystic ovary syndrome. Clin Endocrinol (Oxf). 2012;77(3):343-50.

26. Pal L, Berry A, Coraluzzi L, et al. Therapeutic implications of vitamin D and calcium in overweight women with polycystic ovary syndrome. Gynecol Endocrinol. 2012;28:965-8.

27. Wehr E, Pieber TR, Obermayer-Pietsch B. Effect of vitamin D3 treatment on glucose metabolism and menstrual frequency in polycystic ovary syndrome women: a pilot study. J Endocrinol Invest. 2011;34:757-63.

28. Kauffman RP, Tullar PE, Nipp RD, et al. Serum magnesium concentrations and metabolic variables in polycystic ovary syndrome. Acta Obstet Gynecol Scand. 2011;90:452-8.

29. Sharifi F, Mazloomi S, Hajihosseini R, et al. Serum magnesium concentrations in polycystic ovary syndrome and its association with insulin resistance. Gynecol Endocrinol. 2012;28:7-11.

30. Chakraborty P, Ghosh S, Goswami SK, et al. Altered trace mineral milieu might play an aetiological role in the pathogenesis of polycystic ovary syndrome. Biol Trace Elem Res. 2013;152:9-15.

31. Evans JL, Heymann CJ, Goldfine ID, et al. Pharmacokinetics, tolerability, and fructosamine-lowering effect of a novel, controlled-release formulation of alpha-lipoic acid. Endocr Pract. 2002;8:29-35.

32. Masharani U, Gjerde C, Evans JL, et al. Effects of controlled-release alpha lipoic acid in lean, nondiabetic patients with polycystic ovary syndrome. J Diabetes Sci Technol. 2010;4: 359-64.

33. Cerda C, Pérez-Ayuso RM, Riquelme A, et al. Nonalcoholic fatty liver disease in women with polycystic ovary syndrome. J Hepatol. 2007;47:412-7.

34. Gambarin-Gelwan M, Kinkhabwala SV, Schiano TD, et al. Prevalence of nonalcoholic fatty liver disease in women with polycystic ovary syndrome. Clin Gastroenterol Hepatol. 2007;5:496-501.

35. Alwayn IP, Andersson C, Zauscher B, et al. Omega-3 fatty acids improve hepatic steatosis in a murine model: potential implications for the marginal steatotic liver donor. Transplantation. 2005;79:606-8.

36. Cussons AJ, Watts GF, Mori TA, et al. Omega-3 fatty acid supplementation decreases liver fat content in polycystic ovary syndrome: a randomized controlled trial employing proton magnetic resonance spectroscopy. J Clin Endocrinol Metab. 2009;94:3842-8.

37. Mohammadi E, Rafraf M, Farzadi L, et al. Effects of omega-3 fatty acids supplementation on serum adiponectin levels and some metabolic risk factors in women with polycystic ovary syndrome. Asia Pac J Clin Nutr. 2012;21:511-8.

Adjuvants for Improving Ovarian Reserve in Poor Responders

Mayoukh Kumar Chakraborty, Gautam Khastgir

■ INTRODUCTION

The basis of assisted reproductive technology (ART) is the development of adequate number of follicles and quality of retrieved oocyte. In 21st century, the changes in the social structure have led to delayed childbearing among women after completing their education and professional establishment. Many of these women are in late 30s and 40s obviously have poor ovarian reserve (POR). In addition with the increasing trend of POR even in lesser aged women, the challenge for getting good quality and quantity of oocyte is getting bigger.

Poor ovarian reserve is defined as failure to obtain sufficient number of follicles or obtain inadequate number of oocytes on ovarian stimulation. The diagnostic criteria for poor ovarian responders were laid down by the Bologna criteria in 2011. According to this classification, the women were divided into four categories based on qualitative and quantitative parameters:[1]

1. Age (≥40 years)
2. Antral follicle count (AFC < 5–7)
3. Anti-Müllerian hormone (AMH < 0.5–1.1 ng/mL)
4. Ovarian response to previous stimulation (≤ 3 oocytes with a conventional stimulation).

Subsequently, over the years, the latest criteria being propounded are the Patient-oriented Strategies Encompassing Individualized Oocyte Number (POSEIDON) classification.

■ POOR OVARIAN RESPONSE—AN ENIGMA

For the management of POR, various modalities of management have been proposed over the years, but all have different efficacies or therapeutic response.

A Cochrane review concluded in 2010 that no specific therapy could be stamped with providing the adequate benefit in poor responders.[2]

■ POSEIDON CLASSIFICATION (TABLE 1)

The etiopathogenesis of POR is diverse with multiple underlying causes. The latest POSEIDON classification **(Table 1)** has considered age as vital criteria for aneuploidy rate and ovarian response. Study of this classification on larger sample size is required.

The management of POR is still restricted to limited number of therapeutic modalities as discussed. The efficacy of these agents needs to be researched in more detail.

In this article, a concise review would be made regarding the various modalities of management in poor responders.

TABLE 1: POSEIDON classification.

POSEIDON group 1	POSEIDON group 2
Age < 35 years AFC ≥ 5 AMH ≥ 1.2 ng/mL With an unexpected poor or suboptimal ovarian response *Subgroup 1a <4 oocytes** *Subgroup 1b 4–9 oocytes**	Age > 35 years AFC ≥ 5 AMH ≥ 1.2 ng/mL With an unexpected poor or suboptimal ovarian response *Subgroup 2a <4 oocytes** *Subgroup 2b 4–9 oocytes**
POSEIDON group 3	POSEIDON group 4
Age < 35 years AFC < 5 AMH < 1.2 ng/mL With poor ovarian reserve prestimulation parameters	Age ≥ 35 years AFC < 5 AMH < 1.2 ng/mL With poor ovarian reserve prestimulation parameters

*Retrieved after standard stimulation.
(AFC: antral follicle count; AMH: anti-Müllerian hormone; POSEIDON: Patient-oriented Strategies Encompassing Individualized Oocyte Number)

ANDROGENS

- Dehydroepiandrosterone (DHEA)
- Androstenedione
- Testosterone.

Mechanism of action: Expression of insulin-like growth factor-1 (IGF-1) in the serum, which in turn, leads to improvement in response to gonadotropins. They also modulate ovarian physiology including oocyte and follicle maturation and could have local effects on the endometrium during implantation.[3]

Side effects: Androgenic effects—hair loss, oily skin, and acne. Other effects are increased energy and libido.

Dehydroepiandrosterone

The efficacy of DHEA in POR was first reported by Casson in 2000. In his study, he concluded that overall response to ovulation induction in women with POR improved with DHEA.[4]

Follicular-fluid testosterone (40–80%) during ovarian stimulation is derived from DHEA, which acts as a precursor for testosterone in the follicular fluid. It improves AMH, AFC, peak estradiol (E2), number of oocytes retrieved, number of metaphase II oocytes, and high quality embryos.[3]

The dose of DHEA is 25 mg/day in three divided doses or 75 mg/day. It should be prescribed before taking the patient for *in vitro* fertilization (IVF). The effects of DHEA occur within 2 months and peak 4–5 months of supplementation. It is, therefore, advised to start DHEA for at least 6 weeks prior to IVF.[5]

Dehydroepiandrosterone improves clinical pregnancy rate. However, the effects on oocyte retrieval, implantation, and abortion were not significant. Overall, DHEA supplementation has positive impact in women undergoing IVF/intracytoplasmic sperm injection (ICSI) for POR.[5]

A recent retrospective analysis with adjuvants like DHEA or growth hormone (GH) showed significant improvement in live birth rates when compared to no adjuvant therapy.[6]

Testosterone

It is most commonly used in transdermal form as gel or spray. A dose of 10 mg testosterone gel was applied on external side of thigh for 21 days starting from the first day of menstrual period prior to initiation of ovarian stimulation.[7]

Transdermal testosterone significantly increases live birth rate and reduces the doses of follicle-stimulating hormone (FSH) required. A Cochrane review also concluded that pretreatment with DHEA or testosterone may be associated with improvement in live birth rate, but overall quality of evidence is moderate.[8]

GROWTH HORMONE

Growth hormone plays a very important role in the function of granulosa cells. It promotes ovarian steroidogenesis and follicular development in the ovary. GH supplementation increased serum E2 level on human chorionic gonadotropin (hCG) day, metaphase II oocyte number, two PN number, and obtained embryo number. However, there was no significant difference on clinical pregnancy rate.[9]

Growth hormone-releasing hormones increase the sensitivity of ovaries to gonadotropin stimulation and thereby enhance follicular development. It also enhances the oocyte quality by accelerating and coordinating cytoplasmic maturation. GH-releasing factors may improve pregnancy rates in poor responders. It is started concomitantly with gonadotropins. The dose varies from 4 IU to 8 IU daily or 10–24 IU on alternate days in patients with diminished ovarian reserve.

The use of GH in poor responders has been found to show significant improvement in live birth rates, but it is not clearly evident that which subgroup of women would benefit the most from adjuvant GH.[10] A Cochrane review concluded that the trials of GH were few and with a small sample size. Hence, more robust evidence is required before implementing GH routinely in IVF.[11]

RECOMBINANT LUTEINIZING HORMONE

Luteinizing hormone (LH) maintains the concentrations of intraovarian androgens and as a result promotes steroidogenesis and follicular growth. Numerous studies have validated that poor responders would benefit by adding LH in their stimulation cycles. However, a systematic review and meta-analysis of eight trials in 2014 found no significant benefit by addition of LH in stimulation cycles.[12]

The Efficacy and Safety of Pergoveris in assisted reproductive technology (ESPART) trial concluded that there was improved live birth rate in women with moderate-to-severe POR group.[13] The number of oocytes retrieved was similar following stimulation with either recombinant human FSH (r-hFSH)/recombinant human LH (r-hLH) or r-hFSH monotherapy.[14]

The optimal timing of administration is the midfollicular phase which corresponds with gonadotropin-releasing hormone (GnRH) antagonist administration. The optimal quantitative and qualitative ovarian response and embryo quality were achieved by using rLH (150 IU/day) independently from the total administered dose whereas the total dose had a greater effect than the timing of administration in improving endometrial thickness.[15]

VASOACTIVE SUBSTANCES AND STEROIDS

It has been hypothesized that the use of vasoactive substances increases the ovarian vascularity leading to better delivery of the gonadotropins and ultimately resulting in better folliculogenesis and ovarian response.

Vasoactive substances like aspirin and argiprime have been studied. Some studies have reported beneficial effects of aspirin from the day of embryo transfer. However, some studies have demonstrated that low-dose aspirin and prednisolone did not improve uterine blood flow, implantation, and pregnancy rates.[16] A meta-analysis and a systematic review in 2007 postulated that low-dose aspirin did not increase the clinical pregnancy rate per embryo transfer.[16]

ESTRADIOL IN THE LUTEAL PHASE

The use of estradiol as a priming agent in the luteal phase would improve synchronization of the pool of follicles available to controlled ovarian stimulation. It has been studied that if used with or without GnRH antagonist, it decreases the risk of cycle cancelation and increase chances of clinical pregnancy in poor responders.[17,18] More robust evidence in the form of large randomized controlled trial (RCT) need to be conducted before implementing regularly in poor responders.

FUTURE

We can be hopeful that experimental medicine will make a breakthrough in the management of POR. In-vitro follicle activation is contemplated in poor ovarian responders.[19,20] Autologous mitochondrial transfer to improve the implantation potential and quality of embryo has been studied.[21] Genome of a poor responder can be taken into consideration when designing drugs and planning a treatment protocol. Last but not the least, the use of stem cells is being studied extensively in women with ovarian failure or poor responder.[21,22]

CONCLUSION

No single treatment would be beneficial in the women with POR. Treatment has to be individualized in all steps including choice of GnRH analog, gonadotropin type and dose, ovulation trigger, and finally the choice of adjuvants. More research in this field of POR is required to prepare a standard treatment protocol.

REFERENCES

1. Esteves SC, Roque M, Bedoschi GM, et al. Defining Low Prognosis Patients Undergoing Assisted Reproductive Technology: POSEIDON Criteria—The Why. Front Endocrinol (Lausanne). 2018;9:461.
2. Pandian Z, McTavish AR, Aucott L, et al. Interventions for 'poor responders' to controlled ovarian hyperstimulation (COH) in in-vitro fertilisation (IVF). Cochrane Database Syst Rev. 2010;(1):CD004379.
3. Casson PR, Santoro N, Elkind-Hirsch K, et al. Postmenopausal dehydroepiandrosterone administration increases free insulin-like growth factor-I and decreases high-density lipoprotein: A six-month trial. Fertil Steril. 1998;70:107-10.
4. Casson PR, Lindsay MS, Pisarska MD, et al. Dehydroepiandrosterone supplementation augments ovarian stimulation in poor responders: a case series. Hum Reprod. 2000;15:2129-32.
5. Barad DH, Brill H, Gleicher N. Update on the use of dehydroepiandrosterone supplementation among women with diminished ovarian function. J Assist Reprod Genet. 2007;24:629-34.
6. Keane KN, Hinchliffe PM, Rowlands PK, et al. DHEA supplementation confers no additional benefit to that of growth hormone on pregnancy and live birth rates in IVF patients categorized as poor prognosis. Front Endocrinol (Lausanne). 2018;9:14.
7. González-Comadran M, Durán M, Solà I, et al. Effects of transdermal testosterone in poor responders undergoing IVF: Systematic review and meta-analysis. Reprod Biomed Online. 2012;25:450-9.
8. Nagels HE, Rishworth JR, Siristatidis CS, et al. Androgens (dehydroepiandrosterone or testosterone) for women undergoing assisted reproduction. Cochrane Database Syst Rev. 2015;(11):CD009749.
9. Yu X, Ruan J, He LP, et al. Efficacy of growth hormone supplementation with gonadotrophins in vitro fertilization for poor ovarian responders: An updated meta-analysis. Int J Clin Exp Med. 2015;8:4954-67.
10. Li XL, Wang L, Lv F, et al. The influence of different growth hormone addition protocols to poor ovarian responders on clinical outcomes in controlled ovary stimulation cycles: A systematic review and meta-analysis. Medicine (Baltimore). 2017;96:e6443.
11. Duffy JM, Ahmad G, Mohiyiddeen L, et al. Growth hormone for in vitro fertilization. Cochrane Database Syst Rev. 2010;(1):CD000099.
12. Venetis CA, Kolibianakis S, Bosdou JK, et al. Addition of recombinant LH in poor responders undergoing ovarian stimulation with recombinant FSH and GnRH analogues for in vitro fertilization: A systematic review and meta-analysis. Fertil Steril. 2011;96:57.
13. Humaidan P, Schertz J, Fischer R. Efficacy and safety of pergoveris in assisted reproductive technology—ESPART: Rationale and design of a randomised controlled trial in poor ovarian responders undergoing IVF/ICSI treatment. BMJ Open. 2015;5:e008297.
14. Gizzo S, Andrisani A, Noventa M, et al. Recombinant LH supplementation during IVF cycles with a GnRH-antagonist in estimated poor responders: A cross-matched pilot investigation of the optimal daily dose and timing. Mol Med Rep. 2015;12:4219-29.
15. Revelli A, Dolfin E, Gennarelli G, et al. Low-dose acetylsalicylic acid plus prednisolone as an adjuvant treatment in IVF: A prospective, randomized study. Fertil Steril. 2008;90:1685-91.
16. Gelbaya TA, Kyrgiou M, Li TC, et al. Low-dose aspirin for in vitro fertilization: A systematic review and meta-analysis. Hum Reprod Update. 2007;13:357-64.
17. Reynolds KA, Omurtag KR, Jimenez PT, et al. Cycle cancellation and pregnancy after luteal estradiol priming in women defined

as poor responders: A systematic review and meta-analysis. Hum Reprod. 2013;28:2981-9.

18. Lossl K, Andersen CY, Loft A, et al. Short-term androgen priming by use of aromatase inhibitor and hCG before controlled ovarian stimulation for IVF: A randomized controlled trial. Hum Reprod. 2008;23:1820-9.

19. Zhai J, Yao G, Dong F, et al. In vitro activation of follicles and fresh tissue autotransplantation in primary ovarian insufficiency patients. J Clin Endocrinol Metab. 2016;101:4405-12.

20. Oktay K, Baltaci V, Sonmezer M, et al. Oogonial precursor cell-derived autologous mitochondria injection to improve outcomes in women with multiple IVF failures due to low oocyte quality: A clinical translation. Reprod Sci. 2015;22:1612-7.

21. Morohaku K, Tanimoto R, Sasaki K, et al. Complete in vitro generation of fertile oocytes from mouse primordial germ cells. Proc Natl Acad Sci USA. 2016;113:9021-6.

22. Goyal R. Adjuvant therapy in poor ovarian response—where do we stand? Fertil Sci Res. 2018;5:4-8.

CHAPTER
5

Adjuvants for Improving Uterine Blood Flow

Sunita Tandulwadkar, Seema Pandey

■ INTRODUCTION

Endometrium is one of the integral factors in implantation and pregnancy. Pregnancy rate is affected by endometrial thickness. Several studies have concluded that results of implantation and pregnancy rate are not good if endometrium is too thin or very thick. The minimal thickness of endometrium for getting pregnancy was reported to be 7.0 mm.[1] The reason for this thin endometrium could be due to high blood flow impedance of uterine radial arteries, interestingly this high impedance remains throughout the menstrual cycle in these women and could be responsible for poor endometrial growth and thin endometrium.[2,3] **Flowchart 1** explains the possible mechanism.

We all know that endometrial thickness varies with the vascularity of endometrium and subendometrial area, irrespective of the estrogen and progesterone concentration.

In a retrospective study of 500 ovum donation-embryo transfer cycles published by Nagori and Panchal in 2012, they observed that conception rates were almost doubled when endometrial vascularity was seen in zones 3 and 4 of the endometrium than when it reached only zones 1 and 2 with low abortion rates.[4] Another study done in 2014 by Sardana et al. on 165 women undergoing frozen embryo transfer (FET) cycles also found that the presence of endometrial vascularity significantly improves the outcome in FET cycles.[5]

Though there is no established protocol to treat this condition, but extended estrogen treatment and adjuvant therapy have been used for thin endometrium, but there is not much proven evidence in these treatments.

■ COMMON ADJUVANTS TO INCREASE UTERINE BLOOD FLOW

- Vasodilators—sildenafil citrate
- Pentoxifylline (PTX)
- Vitamin E
- L-arginine
- Low-dose aspirin
- Low-molecular-weight heparin (LMWH)
- Intrauterine perfusion of granulocyte-colony stimulating factor (GCSF)
- Low-dose human chorionic gonadotropin (hCG)
- Platelet-rich plasma (PRP)
- Stem cells
- Acupuncture.

Vasodilators

Vasodilators, by relaxing vascular smooth muscles, increase the flow in uterine artery till radial arteries which

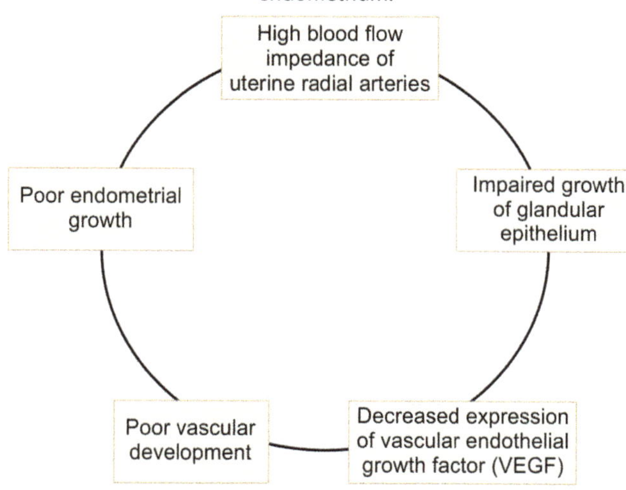

Flowchart 1: Proposed pathophysiological mechanism of thin endometrium.

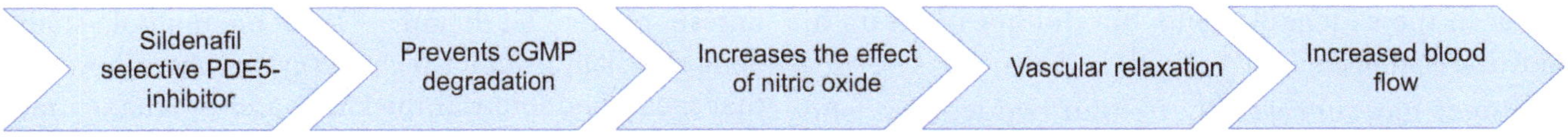

Fig. 1: Mechanism of action of sildenafil citrate.
(cGMP: cyclic guanosine monophosphate; PDE5: phosphodiesterase type 5)

in turn increases the thickness as well as the quality of endometrium. Most commonly used vasodilator is sildenafil citrate, followed by PTX; rest like glyceryl trinitrate (GTN), nifedipine, amlodipine, nimodipine, and isosorbide mononitrate are not in much use because of the side effects.

Functions of Vasodilators in Endometrium

- Smooth muscle relaxation
- Amelioration of endometrial receptivity
- Enhanced endometrial development
- Increased implantation rates.

How do vasodilators work?
- By inhibitory effect on myometrium (in very low dose) (GTN)
- Hydrogen peroxide (H_2O_2) induced damage prevention of embryos (PTX)
- Improves pregnancy rate in thin endometrium patients (PTX + vitamin E)
- Prevention or delay of luteinizing hormone (LH) surge in clomiphene citrate (CC) + intrauterine insemination (IUI) cycles (nimodipine).

A Cochrane meta-analysis done in 2018 included 15 studies with a total of 1,326 women. All included studies compared a vasodilator versus placebo or no treatment. They concluded that there was insufficient evidence for vasodilators to increase live birth rates however, there was low quality evidence in favor of increased clinical pregnancy rates, but moderate evidence was there for increased adverse effects related to the vasodilators and more adequately powered studies are needed.[6]

Sildenafil Citrate

Sildenafil citrate was first studied by Pfizer for the treatment of hypertension and angina pectoris, but the drug did not have any beneficial effect, instead it was found that it could cause penile erections and later Pfizer patented sildenafil for the treatment of erectile dysfunction (ED). Isoforms of nitric oxide synthase are found in the vascular muscles of endometrium and myometrium and that could be the possible basis of its action on endometrium.[7]

Mechanism of action: Sildenafil is a selective type-5 phosphodiesterase inhibitor which augments vasodilatory effect of nitric oxide on vascular smooth muscles by preventing the degradation of cyclic guanosine monophosphate

(cGMP). As a result, there is an improvement in uterine blood flow. If given vaginally in conjunction with estrogen, sildenafil induces the proliferation of endometrium.[8]

Its mechanism of action is increased in uterine artery blood flow and endometrial thickness **(Fig. 1)**.

Additional actions of sildenafil:
- It has been observed in animal studies that sildenafil plays a role in both implantation and decidualization (cellular changes in the endometrium in preparation for implantation of the embryo caused by the effects of progesterone) by affecting $\beta(3)$ integrin (which are cell membrane proteins) and vascular endothelial growth factor (VEGF) expressed during implantation period.
- Improving pregnancy rates and reducing miscarriage rates—studies have shown that vaginal sildenafil has the power of significantly reducing peripheral natural killer (NK) cell activity and therefore, improving pregnancy rates in women with histories of recurrent miscarriages. Although how sildenafil influences NK cell activity is unclear, but effect seems to be by improving uterine artery flow.[9]

In a double-blind randomized study conducted on 15 nonpregnant, nulliparous women, Hale S et al. investigated the effect of sildenafil on uterine volumetric flow (UVF) and vascular impedance. They received either placebo or sildenafil (25 mg or 100 mg) during the luteal phase of the menstrual cycle. At 1 and 3 hours postadministration, color Doppler ultrasound of both uterine arteries was performed at baseline to calculate resistance index (RI) and UVF. Those who received sildenafil showed significantly increased UVF and decreased RI over the 3-hour monitoring period. They concluded that women in the luteal phase, who received sildenafil, demonstrated a significant increase in UVF.[8]

Sildenafil vaginal gel significantly increased endometrial thickness, uterine blood flow, and possibly increase pregnancy rate in anovulatory patients with CC failure due to thin endometrium.[9]

In a randomized controlled trial (RCT) on 80 women, Firouzabadi et al. studied the effect of sildenafil citrate on ultrasonographic ET and its pattern in an FET cycle and found that endometrial thickness and triple line pattern were significantly better in the group who received 50.0 mg of sildenafil twice daily starting from the first day of cycle till the day of starting of progesterone along with estrogen. Implantation rates and chemical pregnancy rates were higher in the sildenafil group, but did not reach up to statistical significance.[10]

Zinger has successfully treated two women who had inadequate endometrium after surgical resection of Asherman's syndrome which had occurred following postpartum curettage leading to secondary infertility. These two women were not conceiving even after surgical correction and medical treatment for subfertility due to thin endometrium. Subsequently, both of them conceived in the first treatment cycle with vaginal sildenafil citrate. On transvaginal ultrasound, endometrial thickness was improved when sildenafil citrate was administered.[11]

Check et al, compared sildenafil with vaginal estradiol in women with thin endometrium. Women failing to attain an 8-mm endometrial thickness on either the oocyte retrieval cycle or their first FET despite an oral graduated E2 regimen were put again on graduated oral E2 and were also randomly assigned to vaginal sildenafil or vaginal E2 therapy. Endometrial thickness was compared between the groups. Neither vaginal estrogen nor sildenafil significantly improved EM or blood flow in the subsequent FET cycle. They concluded that the use of sildenafil may not help all patients with a thin endometrial lining. Women with intractable damage to the basal endometrium are less likely to respond to increased uterine blood flow.[12] Therefore use of sildenafil in women with thin endometrium cannot be taken as a panacea.

Pentoxifylline and Vitamin E

Pentoxifylline and vitamin E in combination have been reported to improve endometrial thickness probably by being anti-inflammatory in action and decreasing tumor necrosis factor-α (TNF-α) levels. Pentoxifylline (PTX) as a derivative of methyl xanthine that inhibits phosphodiesterase and induces vasodilatation. It also mediates inflammatory process and increases phagocytic activity by inhibiting cytokines, which leads to growth of glandular epithelium, blood vessels and VEGF protein expression. Vitamin E or α-Tocopherol, as an antioxidant blocks oxygen free radicals and acts as a vasodilator. Pentoxifylline daily for at least 9 months. This combination was found to improve the endometrial thickness in radiation-induced damage to endometrium which was

unresponsive to E2 therapy.[13] There are multiple studies done especially in donor-recipient cycles where they found that mean endometrial thickness and pregnancy rates increased, but the average duration of treatment was long around 6–8 months. Dosage used varied from 400 mg + 500 IU to 800 mg + 1,000 IU twice a day.

Acharya et al. administered combined PTX and tocopherol (800 mg and 1,000 IU, respectively) to 20 infertile patients with thin endometrium over an average duration of 8.1 months. There was a significant increase in endometrial thickness at the end of the treatment (4.9 mm ± 1.5 mm vs. 7.4 mm ± 0.9 mm, $p = 0.001$) resulting in a 40% pregnancy rate.[14]

L-arginine

The action of L-arginine is at various levels. Arginine plays an important role in vasodilation, activating immune system, and inflammatory process.

Takasaki et al. evaluated its effect on women with a recurrent thin endometrium (6 mg/day). They observed increase in vascular flow of radial uterine arteries in 89% of their patients and endometrial growth greater than 8 mm in 67% of their patients.[15]

Heparin and Low-molecular-weight Heparin

A polysulfated glycosaminoglycan, heparin, interacts with proteins containing positively-charged amino acids while LMWH is derived from heparin by enzymatic chemical depolymerization of unfractionated heparin. Due to high binding affinity of these molecules, they bind to antithrombin, growth factors, and their receptors as well as extracellular matrix. Proteoglycans of heparin sulfate are expressed throughout the genital tract and play an important role in regulation of endometrial cycling. This function of heparin and LMWH in positive modulation of the process of decidualization, implantation, adhesion, and differentiation is represented in **Figure 2**. Apart from its traditional role in inherited and acquired thrombophilia, it works by preventing clotting during implantation and placentation.[16]

In a recent Cochrane review, there was no added value for the use of systemic heparin in *in vitro* fertilization (IVF) cycles, but they proposed studying the possible effects of

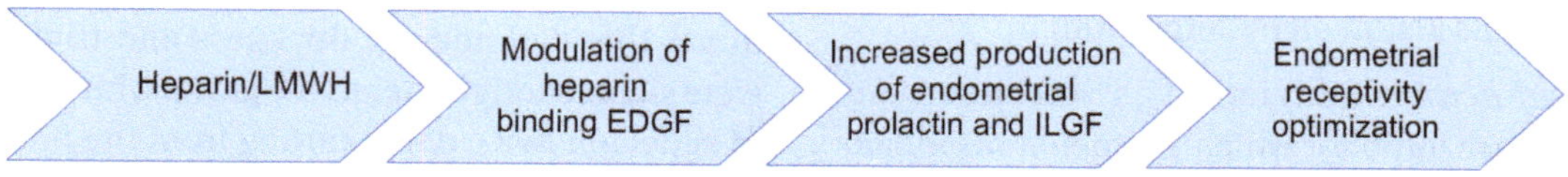

Fig. 2: Mechanism of action of heparin/LMWH.
(EDGF: epidermal growth factor; ILGF: insulin-like growth factor; LMWH: low-molecular-weight heparin)

the intrauterine application of heparin during assisted reproductive technology (ART).[17]

An Egyptian group studied the local effect of LMWH in fresh IVF cycle where patients were divided into two groups. The treatment group was injected with intrauterine LMWH (500 IU) just after ovum pick-up (OPU) (2–5 days prior to ET) while the control group was injected with a similar volume of tissue culture media instead of LMWH. The local intrauterine injection of LMWH using the above described dose and timing proved safe, but showed no benefit and no increase in either implantation or pregnancy rates in intracytoplasmic sperm injection (ICSI) patients.[18]

Low-dose Aspirin

Low-dose aspirin is said to increase endometrial blood flow by decreasing impedance and pulsatility index of uterine artery. There are mixed reviews regarding the use of low-dose aspirin in improving uterine blood flow and most of these studies did not find any difference in the mean thickness when aspirin was used, but many subgroup analysis had shown better pregnancy rates in those who received low-dose aspirin when compared with control group.[19]

Low-dose Human Chorionic Gonadotropin (Systemic or Intrauterine)

Human chorionic gonadotropin is a hormone produced when woman conceives and is probably responsible for embryo implantation. Intrauterine infusion of hCG has been shown to upregulate cytokines known to be involved with implantation. Injection or instillation of hCG into the uterine cavity prior to ET is used to increase the chances of successful implantation by ensuring sufficient levels of hCG at the implantation site. A recent Cochrane review which included 17 RCTs could not arrive at a conclusion due to heterogenecity of studies. In sub-group analysis it was found that intrauterine injection of hCG in the dose of 500 IU on the day of embryo transfer increased the chance of clinical pregnancy and live birth rate in women who underwent cleavage stage transfer.[20]

Adding low-dose hCG during endometrial preparation with E2 was tried to improve endometrium and was found to be effective in improving pregnancy rates.

Intrauterine Granulocyte-colony Stimulating Factor Instillation

Granulocyte-colony stimulating factor is a cytokine secreted by immune cells such as macrophages and is being used as hematopoietic growth factor, but it has been showing effects on many nonhematopoietic tissues including the endometrium. In a meta-analysis, out of the seven reviewed papers, a case report and one retrospective analysis in FET cycles did not demonstrate a positive effect of GCSF on improving endometrial thickness in patients with thin endometrium while another meta-analysis done in 2017 implied its worth in improving pregnancy rate and decreasing cycle cancelation rates. While the use of GCSF seems promising in increasing endometrial thickness and most likely pregnancy rates, but it is expensive and most studies have small sample sizes and did not use a fixed dose or protocol for administration, which makes the interpretation difficult. Larger prospective, randomized, and placebo-controlled trials are therefore needed.[20-22]

Platelet-rich Plasma

Platelet-rich plasma is defined as a plasma fraction of autologous blood with the concentration of platelets four to five times above normal. It has been shown to improve regeneration in various tissues with the expression of several cytokines and growth factors like platelet-derived growth factor (PDGF), transforming growth factor (TGF), VEGF, epidermal growth factor (EGF), fibroblast growth factor (FGF), insulin-like growth factor I, II (IGF I, II), interleukin-8 (IL-8), and connective tissue growth factor (CTGF). These factors can regulate cell migration, attachment, proliferation and differentiation, and promote extracellular matrix accumulation. If used and researched properly, it can prove to be a promising tool.

Chang and colleagues were first people who reported the efficacy of intrauterine infusion of PRP for endometrial growth in women with thin endometrium. In their trial, PRP was infused in five women with thin endometrium with previous poor response to conventional therapy during the FET cycle. The adequate response was reported in all of them and four pregnancies were reported out of five women.[23]

In a comparatively larger patient series, Tandulwadkar and colleagues tested the efficacy of PRP. In their series, intrauterine instillation of PRP was done in 68 women, over 8 months, who had suboptimal endometrial growth and repeated cycle cancelation in previous cycles, in addition to E2 valerate. FET was performed when the optimal endometrial thickness was observed in terms of thickness, appearance, and vascularity. The mean difference of endometrial thickness (5.0 mm vs. 7.22 mm) post-PRP was found to be significantly different. Vascular signal on color Doppler were seen reaching zones 3 and 4 of the endometrium, signifying increase in vascularity. They reported a positive beta-hCG testing in 60.93% of patients, clinical pregnancy rate 45.31% and two missed abortions, three blighted ova and one ectopic gestation, and two biochemical pregnancies. This study concluded that PRP holds promise in treatment of suboptimal ET and vascularity for ET cycles and reduces the financial and psychosocial burden.[24]

Stem Cell Therapy

The most promising evolving treatment modality in refractory endometrium cases seems to be stem cell therapy, as the administration of intrauterine angiogenic endometrial cells improved the endometrial lining of patients with Asherman's syndrome or refractory thin endometrium. Evidence supports the presence of endometrial stem/progenitor cells in the basalis and functionalis layers of the human endometrium. Looking at the tremendous regenerative capacity of the endometrial lining during each menstrual cycle, we can hypothesize that these stem/progenitor cells play an important role in endometrial regeneration. We have got encouraging response from murine models injected with bone marrow mesenchymal stem cells and it restored endometrial thickness to normal after total body irradiation. Bone-marrow derived endothelial progenitors contribute to formation of new blood vessels in the endometrium. In an early human trial, autologous bone marrow-derived stem cells gave promising results in restoring endometrial thickness for more than 6 months in patients with Asherman's syndrome or refractory thin endometrium, with excellent pregnancy rates following, making stem cell therapy a potentially valuable option for patients who fail other established treatment options. The only limitation is that stem cell therapy is invasive requiring a bone marrow biopsy and interventional radiology assistance for injection into the uterine arterioles.[20,25]

Acupuncture

It is a nonpharmacologic therapy with negligible side effects and is beneficial for increasing the success of IVF as per various studies.

How does acupuncture work?
- By modulating neuroendocrine factors
- By increasing the vascularity of uterus and ovaries
- As immunomodulator
- By reducing stress, anxiety, and depression.

Looking at its noninterfering behavior at various systems of body, acupuncture can be used at any stage of infertility treatment and especially ART.

Pelvic floor neuromuscular electrical stimulation (NMES) has been used in patients with thin lining to improve the results and the final outcome was encouraging.[26]

CONCLUSION

In conclusion, treatments that improve uterine radial artery (RA) blood flow seem to be quite beneficial to improve endometrial growth in patients with a thin endometrium. Though, there is not much evidence in therapies being used at present but interventions like stem cell therapy, platelet rich plasma and vasodilators hold some promise if used properly and large multicentric trials are done, till then verdict is still hanging.

REFERENCES

1. El-Toukhy T, Coomarasamy A, Khairy M, et al. The relationship between endometrial thickness and outcome of medicated frozen embryo replacement cycles. Fertil Steril. 2008;89:832-9.
2. Miwa I, Tamura H, Takasaki A, et al. Pathophysiologic features of "thin" endometrium. Fertil Steril. 2009;91:998-1004.
3. Rogers PA, Lederman F, Taylor N. Endometrial microvascular growth in normal and dysfunctional states. Hum Reprod Update. 1998;4:503-38.
4. Nagori C, Panchal S. Endometrial vascularity: its relation to implantation rates. Int J Infertil Fetal Med. 2012;3:48-50.
5. Sardana D, Upadhyay AJ, Deepika K, et al. Correlation of subendometrial-endometrial blood flow assessment by two-dimensional power Doppler with pregnancy outcome in frozen-thawed embryo transfer cycles. J Hum Reprod Sci. 2014;7:130-5.
6. Gutarra-Vilchez RB, Cosp XB, Glujovsky D, et al. Vasodilators for women undergoing fertility treatment. Cochrane Database Syst Rev. 2018;10:CD010001.
7. Benni JM, Patil PA. An overview on sildenafil and female infertility. Indian J Health Sci Biomed Res. 2016;9:131-6.
8. Hale SA, Jones CW, Osol G, et al. Sildenafil increases uterine blood flow in nonpregnant nulliparous women. Reprod Sci. 2010;17:358-65.
9. Fetih AN, Habib DM, Abdelaal II, et al. Adding sildenafil vaginal gel to clomiphene citrate in infertile women with prior clomiphene citrate failure due to thin endometrium: a prospective self-controlled clinical trial. Facts Views Vis Obgyn. 2017;9:21-7.
10. Firouzabadi RD, Davar R, Hojjat F, et al. Effect of sildenafil citrate on endometrial preparation and outcome of frozen-thawed embryo transfer cycles: a randomized clinical trial. Iran J Reprod Med. 2013;11:151-8.
11. Zinger M, Liu JH, Thomas MA. Successful use of vaginal sildenafil citrate in two infertility patients with Asherman's syndrome. J Womens Health (Larchmt). 2006;15:442-4.
12. Check JH, Graziano V, Lee G, et al. Neither sildenafil nor vaginal estradiol improves endometrial thickness in women with thin endometria after taking oral estradiol in graduating dosages. Clin Exp Obstet Gynecol. 2004;31:99-102.
13. Ashraf A, Marzieh A, Mahshid M, et al. Effects of pentoxifylline and vitamin E on pregnancy rate in infertile women treated by ZIFT: a randomized clinical trial. Iran J Reprod Med. 2009;7:175-9.
14. Acharya S, Yasmin E, Balen AH. The use of a combination of pentoxifylline and tocopherol in women with a thin endometrium undergoing assisted conception therapies—a report of 20 cases. Hum Fertil. 2009;12:198-203.
15. Takasaki A, Tamura H, Miwa I, et al. Endometrial Growth and Uterine Blood Flow: A Pilot Study for Improving Endometrial Thickness in the Patients With a Thin Endometrium. Fertil Steril. 2010;93:1851-8.

16. Potdar N, Gelbaya TA, Konje JC, et al. Adjunct low-molecular-weight heparin to improve live birth rate after recurrent implantation failure: a systematic review and meta-analysis. Hum Reprod Update. 2013;19:674-84.

17. Akhtar MA, Sur S, Raine-Fenning N, et al. Heparin for assisted reproduction: summary of a Cochrane review. Fertil Steril. 2015;103:33-4.

18. Kamel AM, El-Faissal Y, Aboulghar M, et al. Does intrauterine injection of low-molecular-weight heparin improve the clinical pregnancy rate in intracytoplasmic sperm injection? Clin Exp Reprod Med. 2016;43:247-52.

19. Usadi RS, Merriam KS. On-label and off-label drug use in the treatment of female infertility. Fertil Steril. 2015;103:583-94.

20. Lensen S, Shreeve N, Barnhart KT, et al. In vitro fertilization add-ons for the endometrium: it doesn't add-up. Fertil Steril. 2019;112:987-93.

21. Eftekhar M, Sayadi M, Arabjahvani F. Transvaginal perfusion of G-CSF for infertile women with thin endometrium in frozen ET program: A non-randomized clinical trial. Iran J Reprod Med. 2014;12:661-6.

22. Xie Y, Zhang T, Tian Z, et al. Efficacy of intrauterine perfusion of granulocyte colony-stimulating factor (G-CSF) for infertile women with thin endometrium: A systematic review and meta-analysis. Am J Reprod Immunol. 2017;78:12701.

23. Chang Y, Li J, Chen Y, et al. Autologous platelet-rich plasma promotes endometrial growth and improves pregnancy outcome during in vitro fertilization. Int J Clin Exp Med. 2015;8:1286-90.

24. Tandulwadkar SR, Naralkar MV, Surana AD, et al. Autologous Intrauterine Platelet-Rich Plasma Instillation for Suboptimal Endometrium in Frozen Embryo Transfer Cycles: A Pilot Study. J Hum Reprod Sci. 2017;10:208-12.

25. Azizi R, Aghebati-Maleki L, Nouri M, et al. Stem Cell Therapy in Asherman Syndrome and Thin Endometrium: Stem Cell-Based Therapy. Biomed Pharmacother. 2018;102:333-43.

26. Djaali W, Abdurrohim K, Helianthi DR. Management of Acupuncture as Adjuvant Therapy for In Vitro Fertilization. Med Acupunct. 2019;31:361-5.

Adjuvants for Endometrial Receptivity/Luteal Phase

N Sanjeeva Reddy, Radha Vembu

INTRODUCTION

The success rate of an assisted reproductive technology (ART) cycle depends on the quality of the embryos, endometrial receptivity, and embryo transfer technique. Endometrial thickness is one of the limiting factors for implantation following embryo transfer in *in vitro* fertilization/intracytoplasmic sperm injection (IVF/ICSI). The use of adjuvants to enhance the endometrial receptivity is increasing.[1]

The aim of an ART clinician is to improve the pregnancy rate (PR) and live birth rate (LBR). So these patients are usually offered many adjuvant therapies. The immune system helps in implantation, establishing receptivity, tolerating the foreign embryo modulating decidual response, epithelial embryo attachment, trophoblast invasion, and placental morphogenesis. Various adjuvants are proposed to improve the immune response.[2,3] These adjuvants are often used to enhance the endometrial thickness (ET). They include:

- Low-dose aspirin
- Heparin
- Human chorionic gonadotropin (hCG)
- L-arginine
- Gonadotropin-releasing hormone (GnRH) agonist
- Pentoxifylline (PTX)
- Vitamin E
- Acupuncture
- Sildenafil
- Corticosteroids
- Granulocyte colony-stimulating factor (G-CSF)
- Stem cells
- Platelet-rich plasma (PRP)
- Endometrial scratching
- Growth hormone (GH).

Thin endometrium is a frustrating challenge to both clinician and patient. It results in lower PR by hypothesis of harmful reactive oxygen species (ROS) or possibly not enough "soil" to sustain the "seed". In thin endometrium, the proximity of ROS-rich basal layer affects the implantation and embryo development.

The cutoff value of thin endometrium is not absolute, but the most widely accepted cutoff is 7 mm. However, it is not the thickness alone, but the endometrial pattern, window of implantation and the vascularity are the prognostic factors for success.

LOW-DOSE ASPIRIN

Aspirin is an antiplatelet agent which enhances prostacyclin synthesis. It irreversibly inhibits the cyclooxygenase enzyme in the platelets and hence prevents thromboxane synthesis. This in turn causes vasodilation and improves blood perfusion and improves the endometrial receptivity for implantation. This effect is seen in the dose of 75–375 mg/day.[4] Low dose is well tolerated and appears to be safe before and during pregnancy.[5]

Studies have shown inconsistent results about the role of aspirin in ART. Tahereh Madani et al. (2019) observed significant improvement in the clinical pregnancy rate (CPR), implantation rate (IR) and LBR in whom short-term aspirin was given. Even though it did not improve the ET, uterine artery pulsatility index (PI) and resistance index (RI), the suboptimal uterine hemodynamics was lower in aspirin-treated group.[6]

Similarly, in a randomized controlled trial (RCT) where low-dose aspirin was started in the midluteal phase of the previous cycle, showed a significant increase in blood flow velocity, ovarian responsiveness, implantation and PRs.[7]

However, Weckstein et al. observed improvement in IR and CPR in aspirin-treated group without demonstrable increase in ET.[8]

A systematic review and meta-analysis of 13 RCTs on the efficacy of low-dose aspirin in IVF/ICSI cycles observed that aspirin in the dose of 100 mg/day improves the PR.[9] However, studies have also shown contradictory findings and have concluded that it could be even harmful.[10] A study by Kim et al. on the role of low-dose aspirin of 100 mg in 264 frozen-thawed embryo transfer (FET) cycles concluded that there is no advantage of aspirin in improving IR and LBR.[11]

The latest Cochrane review (2016) concluded that there is no evidence to favor routine use of aspirin to improve the PR for general population and based on current RCT, there is no evidence of an effect of aspirin on women undergoing ART as there is no single outcome demonstrating a benefit and current evidence does not exclude the possibility of adverse effects.[12]

An updated mini review (2017) concluded that there is no evidence in favor of routine administration of aspirin for IVF patients or in cases with recurrent implantation failure. However, different authors have reported vaginal bleeding as adverse effects. So the current evidence states that aspirin should be offered only in selected cases.[13]

Recent Canadian Fertility and Andrology Society Clinical Practice Guidelines (2019) recommend against the use of aspirin to improve PRs.[14]

HEPARIN

Heparin used in treatment of thromboembolism has been used in the last decade as an adjuvant in ART. It is speculated to improve the intrauterine environment in infertile women by improving decidualization and activation of growth factors like IGF-1, heparin-binding epidermal growth factor (EGF), cytokine expression in endometrium promoting embryo implantation through trophoblast invasion, and proliferation.[15,16] It is administered subcutaneously in the form of unfractionated heparin (5,000 IU once/twice daily) and low-molecular-weight heparin, (enoxaparin 40–60 mg/day SC, dalteparin 5,000 IU–7,500 IU/day SC) latter has increased bioavailability and half-life. It can be started at or after oocyte retrieval or at embryo transfer.

A mini review (2017) concluded that there is insufficient evidence to recommend heparin as an adjuvant therapy. As adverse effects have been reported, there are no firm conclusions regarding its safety profile. Hence, well-designed RCTs are needed to obtain good quality evidence.[13]

HUMAN CHORIONIC GONADOTROPIN

Human chorionic gonadotropin is known to promote trophoblast invasion and peritrophoblastic immune

tolerance. It also supports different stages of implantation by regulating the proteins involved in the procedure.[17] This increases the interaction between the embryo and the endometrium, hence increases the chances of implantation and PR.[18] However, the results are contradictory.

In a RCT (Shiotani et al.), hCG failed to increase the implantation and PR.[19] Assaf et al. did not find any improvement in IR and PR with the administration of recombinant hCG 250 μg on the day of progesterone initiation, day of embryo transfer and 6 days later.[20] A Cochrane systematic review evaluated the effect of intrauterine administration of hCG, reported an improvement in CPR and LBR in cleavage stage transfer with intracervical hCG dose of 500 IU or greater than with no intracervical administration of hCG.[21] Maryam et al. administered 5,000 U hCG intramuscularly on the day of embryo transfer and then every 72 hours till three doses. As half-life of hCG is 24 hours, it is shown that continuous exposure to hCG is required for crosstalk between embryo and endometrium. So single dose of hCG may not be useful.[17] A recent guideline (2019) does not recommend the use of hCG to improve the PR.[14]

L-ARGININE

L-arginine (nitric oxide donor) supplementation improves the uterine blood flow, endometrial receptivity, and implantation and PRs in comparison to a control group in addition; oral L-arginine improves ET on the day of hCG administration.[22] It is given daily in the dose of 16 g, available as sachets.

GONADOTROPIN-RELEASING HORMONE AGONIST

Gonadotropin-releasing hormone agonists have been tried as an adjuvant for luteal phase support especially in patients with thin endometrium (≤7 mm) in a prospective study with 120 patients undergoing IVF with thin endometrium. Triptorelin 0.1 mg or a placebo was given during luteal support on the day of oocyte retrieval, embryo transfer and 3 days after embryo transfer. There was significant increase in ET (6.89 ± 0.24 mm to 8.92 ± 1.6 mm) in study group when compared to control group (6.8 ± 0.26 mm to 7.12 ± 0.45 mm). PR was also significantly higher in the study group (36.6% vs 13.7%, P < 0.01).[23] Recent guidelines (2019) does not recommend the use of GnRH agonists to improve the PR.[14]

PENTOXIFYLLINE AND TOCOPHEROL (VITAMIN E)

Pentoxifylline is a methylxanthine derivative used in treatment of vascular diseases. PTX along with vitamin E is reported to increase the ET in patients with thin endometrium.

This combination was administered in the dose of 400 mg and 500 IU, respectively in donor recipient cycles with thin endometrium (≤6 mm) who did not respond to micronized vaginal estradiol. There was a significant increase in ET by 1.3 mm ± 1 mm after 6 months of treatment. The pregnancy and delivery rates were 33% and 27%, respectively. However, there was no significant difference in ET between those who conceived and those who did not, before or after treatment.[24] The mechanism of action is not clear but it is hypothesized that it inhibits inflammatory reactions and decreases TNF-α levels. The doses of 800 mg and 1,000 IU, respectively have also been tried and have shown improvement in ET.

A recent guideline (2019) does not recommend the use of pentoxifylline and tocopherol to improve the PR.[14]

ACUPUNCTURE, NEUROMUSCULAR ELECTRIC STIMULATION AND ELECTROACUPUNCTURE

Acupuncture is one of the oldest Chinese medicine which has shown improvement in PRs in ART. It is shown to reduce blood flow impedance across uterine artery in patients undergoing IVF. A study comparing the PRs in study and control group showed reduction in uterine artery blood flow impedance without significant increase in PRs.[25]

Transcutaneous electrical acupuncture point stimulation (TEAS), pelvic floor neuromuscular electrical stimulation (NMES) have also been tried to improve the ET in patients with thin endometrium.

SILDENAFIL

Sildenafil citrate is a phosphodiesterase inhibitor which enhances the vasodilatory effect of nitric oxide and hence increases the subendometrial blood flow. It is given in the dose of 25 mg 6–8 hourly by vaginal route during controlled ovarian stimulation or during HRT in FET cycles. These patients treated with vaginal sildenafil had improvement in ET and decrease in PI. It also improved the PI and PR.[26] Recent guidelines (2019) suggests that there is insufficient evidence to recommend the use of sildenafil to improve PR.[14]

CORTICOSTEROIDS

The uterine receptivity is controlled by natural killer cells (NK cells) and cytokines. So defective cytokine network or excess NK cells can lead to implantation failure and recurrent miscarriages.

Corticosteroids produced in adrenal cortex have potent anti-inflammatory and anti-immunosuppressive properties.

Glucocorticoids have been proposed to improve the IR after ART and protect against miscarriage by acting as immune modulators to reduce NK cells to normal range, normalize the cytokine expression profile in the endometrium and by suppressing endometrial inflammation.[27]

A variety of drugs are available namely prednisolone, methylprednisolone, dexamethasone, and hydrocortisone. The Cochrane review (2012) investigated the use of glucocorticoids around the time of implantation. Among the 14 studies included, they found no evidence of improvement in LBRs [odds ratio (OR) 1.21, 95% confidence interval (CI) 0.67–2.19]. There was no improvement in PRs also (OR 1.16, 95% CI 0.94–1.44). But borderline statistical significance of increased PR in IVF and not ICSI (OR 1.50, 95% CI 1.05–2.13). These findings cannot be extrapolated to patients with autoantibodies, RIF, and unexplained infertility.[28]

In women with recurrent miscarriage, prednisolone decreases the expression of angiogenic factors and decrease the vessel maturation. Corticosteroids along with low-dose aspirin might improve PR after IVF. Excess usage of glucocorticoids in pregnancy can cause adverse effects in placenta, fetal growth restriction, and altered fetal development. It can increase the risk of hypertension, diabetes mellitus, and premature birth. However, long-term studies are required to elucidate the possible cardiometabolic and neuroendocrine development. Prednisolone is category D drug according to food and drug administration (FDA). So routine administration is not indicated.

There are no recommendations for routine use of corticosteroids among unselected women undergoing ART. So well-designed RCTs are required to elucidate which specific groups of women will be benefited.[13]

GRANULOCYTE COLONY-STIMULATING FACTOR

Granulocyte colony-stimulating factor has a direct role in promoting endometrial growth. It is administered intrauterine in the dose of 300 µg 2–9 days before embryo transfer. It is known to increase the ET. In a pilot study, patients with ET < 7 mm on the day of hCG trigger received 300 µg of G-CSF intrauterine infusion 6–12 hours of hCG trigger. A second infusion was given if required. ET increased from 6.4 ± 1.4 mm to 9.3 ± 2.1 mm (P < 0.001) after G-CSF infusion but did not differ between those who conceived and those who did not. The overall PR was 19.1%.[29] In a retrospective study by Li et al. G-CSF (100 µg) intrauterine infusion was administered in patients with ET < 7 mm on the day of ovulation or progesterone start or the day of hCG administration. The cycle cancellation rate due to thin endometrium was lowest in G-CSF group with better IR and CPR.[30]

Granulocyte colony-stimulating factor (300 µg/mL) has also been tried in all patients undergoing IVF or FET regardless of ET in the study group and saline in control group. It was observed that the ET was significantly more by 1.36 mm but with similar CPR.[31]

A recent 2019 guideline does not recommend the use of G-CSF to improve the PR in thin endometrium.[14]

STEM CELL THERAPY

This was first tried in humans in 2011. The basalis and functionalis layer of endometrium shows the presence of endometrial stem/progenitor cells. In addition, hematopoietic and nonhematopoietic bone marrow-derived stem cells (BMDSCs) are recruited to the endometrium in response to injury, these cells along with CD 45+ hematopoietic progenitor cells play a role in the regeneration of endometrium. This has been tried in Asherman's syndrome.

In a human pilot study, autologous CD 133+ BMDSCs was infused into the spiral arterioles of patients with refractory Asherman's syndrome and endometrial atrophy. An increase in ET lasting up to 6 months was seen (4.3–6.7 mm) in Asherman's syndrome, (4.2–5.7 mm) in refractory atrophic endometrium. There were three spontaneous pregnancies and seven pregnancies after embryo transfer.[32] However, recent guidelines (2019) does not recommend the use of stem cells to improve the PR.[14]

PLATELET-RICH PLASMA

Platelet-rich plasma is an autologous source of many factors and substances like PDGF, TGF-β. This helps in regeneration of the tissues. It is administered as 1 mL intrauterine infusion using a catheter. PRP administration as an adjuvant in endometrial preparation in patients with refractory endometrium showed improvement in ET, clinical pregnancy and LBR. It is easy to obtain, autologous, nontoxic, cost-effective with high concentration of growth factors.[33] But, the recent guidelines (2019) does not recommend the use of PRP to improve the PR.[14]

ENDOMETRIAL SCRATCHING

The rationale behind this is the mechanical manipulation of the endometrium induces secretion of several proimplantation chemical factors including cytokines, LIF, IL-11, heparin-binding EGF and this stimulates a better decidual reaction.[34] A single sampling in the proliferative phase is found adequate to improve the reproductive outcome. However, studies are showing contradictory results. A Cochrane review (2015) showed that the endometrial injury between Day 7 of the previous cycle and Day 7 of ET cycle showed an increase in LBR or ongoing PR and CPR in women with previous implantation failure. There was no evidence of any effect on miscarriage as it was low quality evidence.[35]

In a recent RCT (2019) of 1,364 women, endometrial scratch did not show any significant difference in ongoing PRs, CPRs, multiple pregnancy, ectopic pregnancy or miscarriage and they concluded that endometrial scratch did not result in a higher LBR in women undergoing IVF.[36]

GROWTH HORMONE

Low dose of recombinant human growth hormone (rhGH) has been supplemented in patients with thin endometrium. It might improve the endometrial receptivity through blood flow or at molecular level. It might regulate cytokines produced by the uterus, enhancing endometrial receptivity by controlling the expression of adhesion and anti-adhesion proteins. It has been tried in the dose of 4–5 IU every alternate day subcutaneously from the day of progesterone administration till the day of embryo transfer. rhGH might improve the clinical outcomes of FET in patients with thin endometrium between 30 years and 34 years of age. A relatively lower dose for shorter duration would be more safe and cost-effective.[37]

CONCLUSION

The quality of scientific evidence on safety and efficacy of adjuvants to improve LBR is low. Although some adjuvants may have a promising future, large well-designed studies are required to elucidate which subgroup will be benefited.

REFERENCES

1. Gilboa Y, Bar-Hava I, Fisch B, et al. Does intravaginal probiotic supplementation increase the pregnancy rate in IVF–ET cycles? Reprod Biomed Online. 2005;1:71-5.
2. Van Mourik MS, Macklon NS, Heijnen CJ. Embryonic implantation: cytokines, adhesion molecules, and immune cells in establishing an implantation environment. J Leukoc Biol. 2009;85:4-19.
3. Robertson SA. Immune regulation of conception and embryo implantation-all about quality control? J Reprod Immunol. 2010;85:51-7.
4. Dirckx K, Cabri P, Merien A, et al. Does low-dose aspirin improve pregnancy rate in IVF/ICSI? A randomized double-blind placebo controlled trial. Hum Reprod. 2009;24:856-60.
5. Ahrens KA, Silver RM, Mumford SL, et al. Complications and safety of preconception low-dose aspirin among women with prior pregnancy losses. Obstet Gynecol. 2016;127:689-98.
6. Madani T, Ahmadi F, Jahangiri N, et al. Does low-dose aspirin improve pregnancy rate in women undergoing frozen-thawed embryo transfer cycle? A pilot double-blind, randomized placebo-controlled trial. J Obstet Gynaecol Res. 2019;45:156-63.

7. Rubinstein M, Marazzi A, Polak de Fried E. Low-dose aspirin treatment improves ovarian responsiveness, uterine and ovarian blood flow velocity, implantation, and pregnancy rates in patients undergoing in vitro fertilization: a prospective, randomized, double-blind placebo-controlled assay. Fertil Steril. 1999;71:825-9.

8. Weckstein LN, Jacobson A, Galen D, et al. Low-dose aspirin for oocyte donation recipients with a thin endometrium: prospective, randomized study. Fertil Steril. 1997;68:927-30.

9. Wang L, Huang X, Li X, et al. Efficacy evaluation of low-dose aspirin in IVF/ICSI patients evidence from 13 RCTs: A systematic review and meta-analysis. Medicine (Baltimore). 2017;96:e7720.

10. Check JH, Dietterich C, Lurie D, et al. A matched study to determine whether low-dose aspirin without heparin improves pregnancy rates following frozen embryo transfer and/or affects endometrial sonographic parameters. J Assist Reprod Genet. 1998;15:579-82.

11. Kim MJ, Lee HJ, Yu Y, et al. Effect of Low-dose aspirin on implantation and pregnancy rates in patients undergoing frozen-thawed embryo transfer. Korean J Fertil Steril. 2005;32:243-52.

12. Siristatidis CS, Basios G, Pergialiotis V, et al. Aspirin for in vitro fertilisation. Cochrane Database Syst Rev. 2016;11:CD004832.

13. Fabozzi G, Giannini A, Placentino Piscitelli V, et al. Adjuvants therapies for women undergoing IVF: Is there any evidence of their safety and efficacy? An updated mini-review. Obstet Gynecol Int J. 2017;7:00254

14. Liu KE, Hartman M, Hartman A. Management of thin endometrium in assisted reproduction: a clinical practice guideline from the Canadian Fertility and Andrology Society. Reprod Biomed Online. 2019;39:49-62.

15. Potdar N, Gelbaya TA, Konje JC, et al. Adjunct low-molecular-weight heparin to improve live birth rate after recurrent implantation failure: a systematic review and meta-analysis. Hum Reprod Update. 2013;19:674-84.

16. Nelson SM, Greer IA. The potential role of heparin in assisted conception. Hum Reprod Update. 2008;14:623-45.

17. Racicot K, Kwon JY, Aldo P, et al. Understanding the complexity of the immune system during pregnancy. Am J Reprod Immunol. 2014;72:107-16.

18. Eftekhar M, Dashti S, Omidi M, et al. Does luteal phase support by human chorionic gonadotropin improve pregnancy outcomes in frozen-thawed embryo transfer cycles? Middle East Fertil Soc J. 2018;23:300-2.

19. Shiotani M, Matsumoto Y, Okamoto E, et al. Is human chorionic gonadotropin supplementation beneficial for frozen and thawed embryo transfer in estrogen/progesterone replacement cycles?: A randomized clinical trial. Reprod Med Biol. 2017;16:166-9.

20. Ben-Meir A, Aboo-Dia M, Revel A, et al. The benefit of human chorionic gonadotropin supplementation throughout the secretory phase of frozen-thawed embryo transfer cycles. Fertil Steril. 2010;93:351-4.

21. Craciunas L, Tsampras N, Raine-Fenning N, et al. Intrauterine administration of human chorionic gonadotropin (hCG) for subfertile women undergoing assisted reproduction. Cochrane Database Syst Rev. 2018;10:CD011537.

22. Chwalisz K, Garfield RE. Role of nitric oxide in implantation and menstruation. Hum Reprod. 2000;3:96-111.

23. Qublan H, Amarin Z, Al-Qudah M, et al. Luteal phase support with GnRH-a improves implantation and pregnancy rates in IVF cycles with thin endometrium of <or = 7 mm on day of egg retrieval. Hum Fertil (Camb). 2008;11:43-7.

24. Lédée-Bataille N, Olivennes F, Lefaix JL, et al. Combined treatment by pentoxifylline and tocopherol for recipient women with a thin endometrium enrolled in an oocyte donation programme. Hum Reprod. 2002;17:1249-53.

25. Ho M, Huang LC, Chang YY, et al. Electroacupuncture reduces uterine artery blood flow impedance in infertile women. Taiwan J Obstet Gynecol. 2009;48:148-51.

26. Eid ME. Sildenafil improves implantation rate in women with a thin endometrium secondary to improvement of uterine blood flow; "pilot study". Fertil Steril. 2015;104:e342.

27. Krigstein M, Sacks G. Prednisolone for repeated implantation failure associated with high natural killer cell levels. J Obstet Gynaecol. 2012;32:518-9.

28. Nastri CO, Lensen SF, Gibreel A, et al. Endometrial injury in women undergoing assisted reproductive techniques. Cochrane Database Syst Rev. 2012(7):CD009517.

29. Gleicher N, Kim A, Michaeli T, et al. A pilot cohort study of granulocyte colony-stimulating factor in the treatment of unresponsive thin endometrium resistant to standard therapies. Hum Reprod. 2013;28:172-7.

30. Li Y, Pan P, Chen X, et al. Granulocyte colony-stimulating factor administration for infertile women with thin endometrium in frozen embryo transfer program. Reprod Sci. 2014;21:381-5.

31. Barad DH, Yu Y, Kushnir VA, et al. A randomized clinical trial of endometrial perfusion with granulocyte colony-stimulating factor in in vitro fertilization cycles: impact on endometrial thickness and clinical pregnancy rates. Fertil Steril. 2014;101:710-5.

32. Santamaria X, Cabanillas S, Cervello I, et al. Autologous cell therapy with CD133+ bone marrow-derived stem cells from refractory Asherman's syndrome and endometrial atrophy: a pilot cohort study. Hum Reprod. 2016;31:1087-96.

33. Molina A, Sánchez J, Sánchez W, et al. Platelet-rich plasma as an adjuvant in the endometrial preparation of patients with refractory endometrium. JBRA Assist Reprod. 2018;22:42-8

34. Almog B, Shalom-Paz E, Dufort D, et al. Promoting implantation by local injury to the endometrium. Fertil Steril. 2010;94:2026-9.

35. Nastri CO, Lensen SF, Gibreel A, et al. Endometrial injury in women undergoing assisted reproductive techniques. Cochrane Database Syst Rev. 2015;(3):CD009517.

36. Lensen S, Osavlyuk D, Armstrong S, et al. A randomized trial of endometrial scratching before in vitro fertilization. N Engl J Med. 2019;380:325-34.

37. Yang JY, Li H, Lu N, et al. Influence of growth hormone supplementation in patients with thin endometrium undergoing frozen embryo transfer. Reprod Dev Med. 2019;3:49-53.

Adjuvants for Improving the Implantation Potential of the Embryo

Sonal Sagar Vaidya, Swati Sandipan Ingale, Dimple Atul Desai

■ INTRODUCTION

The prevalence of infertility globally is on the rise with at least 50 million couples experiencing infertility. The International Committee for Monitoring Assisted Reproductive Technology (ICMART)'s annual collection of global *in vitro* fertilization (IVF) data has estimated that since 1978, over 8 million babies have been born through the use of IVF globally (1991–2014).[1]

Extensive research in order to understand the intrinsic complexities of a developing embryo with its surroundings has led to development of specifically designed cleanrooms, incubators, culture systems that best mimic the *in vivo* environment.

IVF protocols can be targeted to overcome individualized fertility difficulties. Areas open to manipulation include ovarian stimulation, oocyte collection, and fertilization, with the final stage being the embryo transfer. The success of the embryo transfer is determined largely by the embryo quality and the endometrial receptivity.

Various pharmacological agents, newer technologies, and techniques have been introduced to increase the success rate of assisted reproductive technology (ART). Of these newly introduced adjuvants, some have become the norm, some have proved useless, and others still remain debatable.

In a bid to establish a balance between the "acceptable" live birth rate (LBR) and reducing twinning rate and subsequent obstetrical complication, the IVF centers worldwide are moving toward the elective single embryo transfer (eSET), thereby mandating the need to identify and select the most viable, euploid embryo for transfer.

The adjuvants or the "adjuncts" in the IVF laboratory are meant to maximize the implantation potential of the embryo. These may be an "add-ons" in the culture systems itself, or can be a specific technique. The adjuvants currently deployed within the IVF programs range from gamete selection to the embryo selection and are broadly categorized as invasive or noninvasive.

The understanding of the affordability of these "add-ons", the validity of the treatments offered, their safety and efficacy as well as the current regulations will be the focus of this chapter.

■ SPERM FERTILITY

The contribution of the sperm during fertilization and its profound effects on the embryonic development is well established. This necessitates the real-time selection of the most competent sperm for fertilization in IVF programs. The impact of use of intracytoplasmic morphologically selected sperm injection (IMSI), physiological intracytoplasmic sperm injection (PICSI), and sperm deoxyribonucleic acid fragmentation indices (DFI) has been discussed here.

Intracytoplasmic Morphologically Selected Sperm Injection

Intracytoplasmic morphologically selected sperm injection is an advanced sperm selection technique by which spermatozoa are selected for ICSI after examining them under high magnification (over 6600X) **(Figs. 1A to C)**, as compared to the routine magnification of 200–400X.

Meta-analysis of randomized studies comparing IMSI to intracytoplasmic sperm injection (ICSI) has not shown any difference in LBR and miscarriage rate. Meta-analysis of observational studies, which must be interpreted with caution, revealed an increased LBR and decreased miscarriage rate with IMSI versus ICSI.[2]

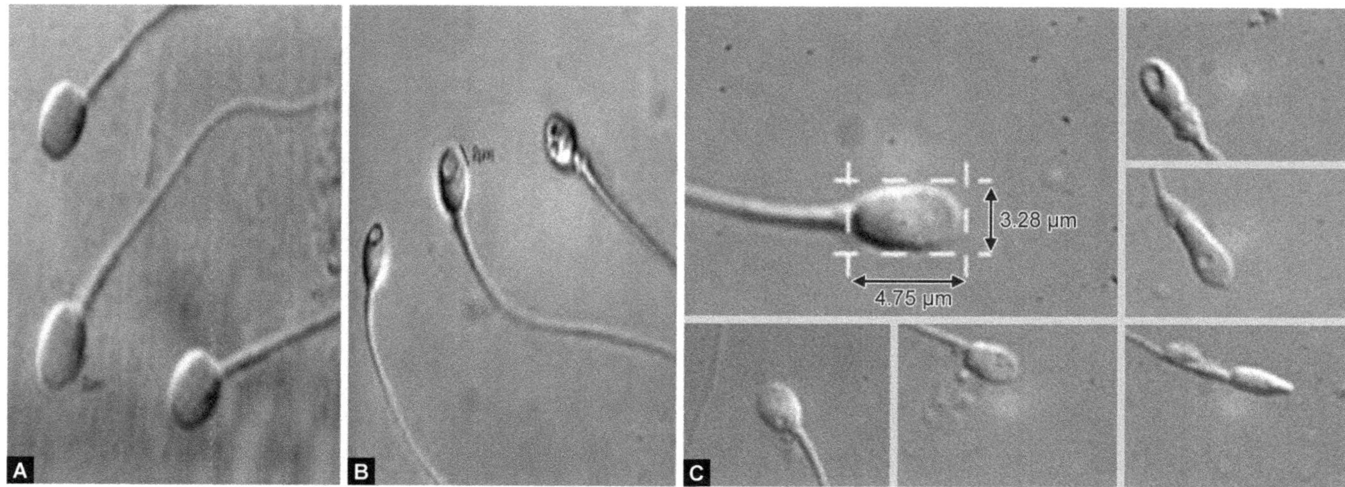

Figs. 1A to C: (A) Normal spermatozoa; (B) Vacuolated spermatozoa; (C) Comparison of different spermatozoa heads with normal head dimensions.

Data analysis demonstrated significant difference in the fertilization rate between IMSI and previous ICSI attempts of these patients (30% vs 52%; P < 0.05). The embryo quality, implantation and pregnancy rates (PRs) with IMSI were also significantly higher than those of their previous ICSI cycles (32% vs 56.4%; 30.2% vs 68.5%; 0.0% vs 62.4%; P < 0.05). The authors concluded that the IMSI procedure improved embryo development and the clinical outcomes in the same infertile couples with male infertility and poor embryo development over their previous ICSI attempts and can be taken up as the treatment of choice in cases of severe male factor (SMF) infertility.[3]

Initial studies have shown that IMSI, using spermatozoa selected under high magnification, is associated with higher PRs in couples with repeated implantation failures.

However, ICSI introduction seemed to have decreased the importance of sperm morphology in assisted reproduction, since fertilization, embryo development, pregnancies, and healthy deliveries can be achieved even in case of severe morphological impairments **(Fig. 2)**.

Meta-analysis results demonstrated no significant difference in fertilization rate between ICSI and IMSI. However, a significantly improved implantation and PR was observed in IMSI cycles. Moreover, the results showed a significantly decreased miscarriage rate in IMSI cycles as compared with ICSI cycles.[4] The presence of nuclear vacuoles in sperm seems to influence embryo development and more specifically blastocyst formation.

The use of high magnification for morphological sperm selection prior to ICSI has been associated with higher PRs and lower miscarriage rates. However there have been studies showing no significant results inclying in favor of IMSI.[5] IMSI instead of ICSI does not have much beneficial effects in the first ART attempts. Patients with severe

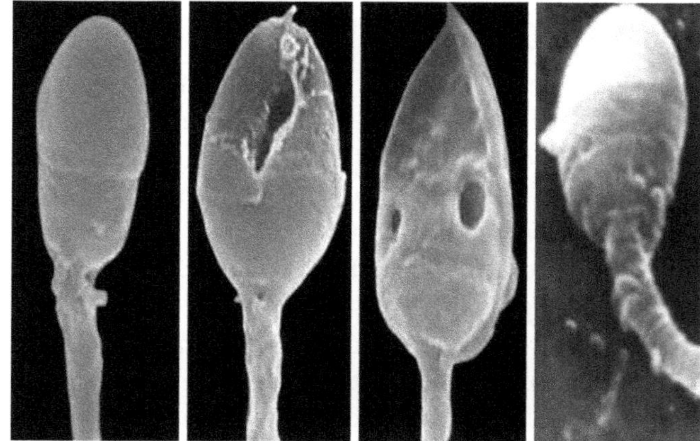

Fig. 2: Severe morphological impairments: Intracytoplasmic morphologically selected sperm injection (IMSI).

teratozoospermia, high DNA fragmentation, and previous ICSI failure should be considered for IMSI.[6]

Classification of spermatozoa selected at 6000X magnification into three different categories: Class I—spermatozoa of good quality, Class II—spermatozoa of poor quality, and Class III—spermatozoa of worse quality **(Figs. 3A to I)**.[7]

Strict morphology is an excellent biomarker of sperm fertilizing capacity, independent of motility and concentration. The head effects or disorders of nuclear membrane and the acrosomal cap and also the disorganization of the chromatin leads to dysfunctional sperm oocyte recognition, binding and fusion with oolemma. DNA fragmentation increases vacuoles which negatively influence embryo development. There is no difference observed between ICSI/IMSI as a function of DFI percentage. However, the rate of DNA fragmentation was low and thus cannot exclude a beneficial effect of IMSI in cases with high DNA fragmentation levels. IMSI shows

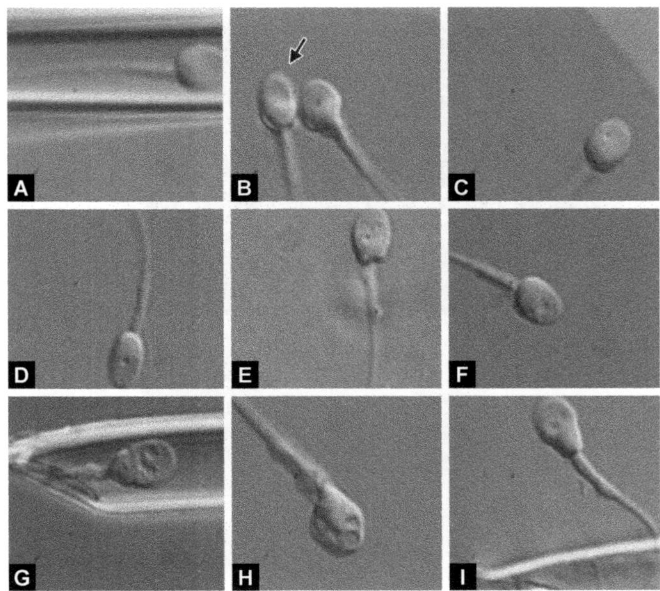

Figs. 3A to I: Classification of spermatozoa selected at 6000X magnification into three different categories: (A to C) Spermatozoa of Class I; (D to F) Spermatozoa of Class II; (G to I) Spermatozoa of Class III.[8]

reduction in miscarriage rates (50%) and higher rates of ongoing pregnancy and live birth.[7] Though it does not signify improved clinical outcome compared to ICSI.

Physiological Intracytoplasmic Sperm Injection

It has been proposed that there is an increase in the rate of aneuploidy in immature spermatozoa. Hyaluronic acid (HA) binding ability is considered to be an indicator of sperm maturity. The HA receptor in mature spermatozoa identified by the HA binding sites of the PICSI dish helps to identify the mature spermatozoa thereby reducing the chromosomal disomy and diploidy.[9]

In HA-selected spermatozoa the frequency of chromosomal disomy and diploidy is reduced four- to sixfold compared with semen sperm fractions. This reduction is similar to the increase in numerical chromosomal aberrations in ICSI children.[9]

When compared PICSI with ICSI in a recent systemic review, it showed no statistically significant difference between the PICSI and the ICSI techniques, for any of the studied outcome measures: live births, clinical pregnancy, implantation, embryo quality, fertilization, and miscarriage rates.[10]

Hyaluronic binding assay (HBA Score) could be used for sperm selection to reduce genetic complications.[11]

Physiological intracytoplasmic sperm injection offered no clear advantage in relation to the full-term live birth. PICSI led to a reduced miscarriage risk but had no effect on clinical pregnancy rate (CPR) or preterm LBR.[12]

Cochrane reviews including two randomized controlled trials (RCTs) on PICSI and nine RCTs on IMSI failed to find any improvement in CPRs when these methods are compared with standard ICSI.[13] However, the multicenter RCT that compared PICSI with standard ICSI found a 12% rise in CPRs with PICSI, which is clinically significant.[14] This RCT also found a significant reduction of pregnancy loss in the PICSI group.

Evidence on PICSI is still in the formative stage and, with limited experience, no serious additional risk (over ICSI) has been reported yet. It may be sensible to recommend PICSI in indicated cases and after careful counseling.

Sperm DNA Fragmentation

Sperm DNA damage has been known to be caused by the oxidative stress to the sperms. The sperm DNA is packaged in highly condensed form with DNA in mature sperm being 85% protamine bound while 15% remains histone bound.[15] It has also been shown that the infertile men show higher histone: protamine ratio than fertile men and the majority of DNA damage is associated with ROS.[16]

The DFI literature has also reported negative impact of sperm DNA fragmentation on the chances of conception irrespective of whether the couple is trying naturally[17-20] or through treatments like IUI,[21,22] IVF1,[4,13,23,24] ICSI.[25-27] The inverse relationship between sperm DNA damage and the fertilization rate for each procedure was stronger in IVF (59% or 19 of 32) than in ICSI (24% or 10 or 42) or IVF and ICSI (33% or 6 of 18) by Simon et al.[28]

DNA fragmentation: Tests can be classified as:

- *Direct assays:*
    - *TUNEL (terminal deoxynucleotidyl transferase mediated deoxyuridine triphosphate-nick-end labeling) assay* (single strand break and double strand break), quantifies the incorporation of fluorescent deoxyuridine triphosphate (dUTP) **(Fig. 4A)**.
    - *ISNT (in situ nick translation)*: This is basically for single strand breaks and known as modified TUNEL. It includes the incorporation of biotinylated-dUTP at the ssDNA in a reaction. This reaction is catalyzed by template dependent enzyme DNA polymerase-1.
    - *Comet assay* at neutral pH (sdSB) (single-cell gel electrophoresis) **(Fig. 4B)**.
- *Indirect assays: (Denaturation of DNA)*
    - *SCSA (sperm chromatin structure assay)*: Denaturation of DNA followed by staining with AO is a flow-cytometric method, measures the metachromatic shift of acridine orange (AO) fluorescence from green to red—green (native DNA) and red (denatured DNA) **(Fig. 4C)**.

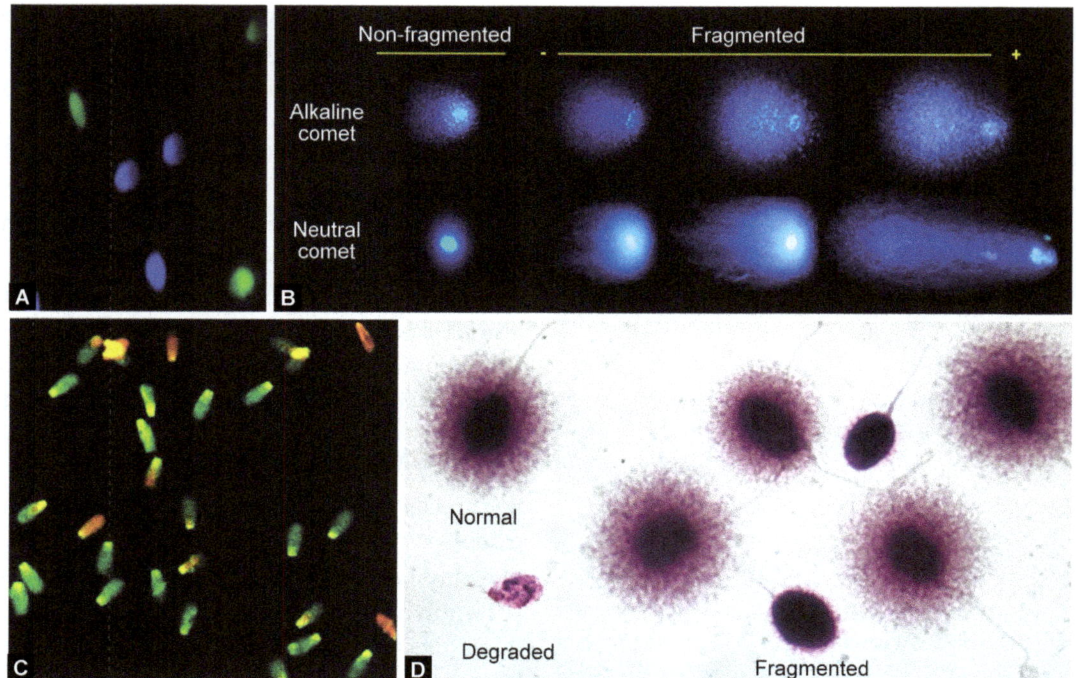

Figs. 4A to D: (A) TUNEL assay—sperm in green indicated DNA fragmentation;[29] (B) Comet assay;[30] (C) Sperm chromatin structure assay (SCSA);[31] (D) Sperm chromatin dispersion (SCD) test.[32]

- *SCD (sperm chromatin dispersion) test* is based on the principle that sperm with fragmented DNA fail to produce the dispersed DNA loops after acidic denaturation (halos) while the normal sperm produce a halo **(Fig. 4D)**.

The important questions about all these methods are whether they reveal the same type of damage, whether they obtain comparable results and last but not least, whether they are standardized.[33]

However, some meta-analysis had no significant difference between the groups with high sperm DNA damage when compared with the group with low sperm DNA damage.[24,25,34]

Highly conflicting results of sperm DNA damage on fertilization outcomes and impact on pregnancy in current scenario has resulted in the exclusion of this test in a routine IVF practice. Hence, though this test being noninvasive diagnostic test and involving no risk to the patient, Human Fertilization and Embryology Authority (HFEA) has given no rating to this adjuvant.

■ CULTURE MEDIA

The culture media is under continuous development and scrutiny with the hope of maximizing the developmental potential of the embryos *in vitro*. Culture media are stringently controlled for the components and their purity. Amino acids, salts/ions, lipids, energy substrates, vitamins, antibiotics, antioxidants, human serum albumin (HSA),

pH stabilizers, surfactants are commonly added to the culture media.[35] Some of these components namely the HSA are largely undefined while some components have unclear effects on the developing embryo. Additionally, culture media with HA (discussed later) or GM-CSF— recombinant human cytokine granulocyte-macrophage colony stimulating factor[36] are also available commercially. Adherence compounds are added to the embryo transfer medium to improve the PRs in many ART centers. Mostly hyaluronan and in some studies fibrin sealant and protein supplements have been tried.

The latest Cochrane review of 3,898 participants from 17 RCTs demonstrated moderate quality evidence for an improvement in CPR and LBR, with an associated increase in multiple PR, when transfer medium was supplemented with HA.[37] More recent RCT by Fancsovits et al. (2015)[38] looked at 581 cycles and did not show a benefit in implantation rate (IR), CPR or LBR, but found a higher birth weight in the HA group. Hyaluronan-enriched transfer medium (HETM) can improve the embryo IRs and CPRs in patients with repeated implantation failure in the third or more frozen-thawed embryo transfer (FET) attempt. However, the use of HETM for first and second FET should be done with caution.[39]

Granulocyte-macrophage colony-stimulating factor is a cytokine/growth factor produced by the epithelial cells in the human uterus and oviducts, in presence of estrogen. It is shown to enhance the embryonic growth and viability by exerting positive control on various paths such as cell proliferation, blastocyst formation, hatching as well as implantation.[40,41] The beneficial nature of GM-CSF in terms of CPRs has yet to be resolved, although there is good evidence for women with more than one miscarriage but the study size is small and effect on epigenetics is still unclear. GM-CSF shows significant increase in ongoing pregnancy rates and live birth rates.[42]

Large offspring syndrome, errors in methylation and effects on epigenome are serious concerns[39,43] and hence full revelation of the media components is necessary.[40] Caution should be practiced while adding growth factors and hormones to the culture media.

◼ COCULTURE

Autologous endometrial coculture has been suggested to improve the embryo quality by providing increased levels of insulin-like growth factor-I (IGF-I), IGF-II, vascular endothelial growth factor-A (VEGF-A), and VEGF-C in the culture system thereby providing the natural uterine environment.[44]

A recent study from Indian Journal of Medical Research demonstrated beneficial role of cumulus cells coculture technique in embryonic development in women undergoing IVF using donor oocytes fertilized by ICSI. This study showed that a simple, low-cost and nonlaborious cumulus cell coculture system could result in improved IRs and clinical pregnancy rates (CPRs) during IVF.[45]

Data from another study suggest that the use of coculture exploiting the patient's own endometrial cells could favor the development of embryos into good-quality blastocysts and may be specifically beneficial to freeze-all cycles. While several teams have concentrated their works more specifically on patients with IVF failure,[46-48] data from this study suggest that all patients could benefit from AECC. However, a confirmatory study using patients as the denominator rather than embryos would help to confirm this proposal, as well as a follow-up of children born as a result of these treatments.[49]

◼ ARTIFICIAL OOCYTE ACTIVATION

Fertilization failure is often encountered in patients undergoing IVF. Both sperm and oocyte can cause failed activation. Though its occurrence is less in ICSI cycles, it is not rare. Artificial oocyte activation (AOA) is proposed to overcome the fertilization failure by using calcium ionophore and few other substances like strontium chloride and calcimycin.[50]

The couples with poor fertilization rates have better results with calcium ionophore treatment. It improves cleavage rates, IRs, PRs, and live birth rates.[51]

Human oocytes activation involves the cascade of event which leads to formation of male and female pronuclei and progression in first embryonic cell cycle. Oocyte activation is characterized by a dramatic rise in intracellular calcium concentration, which in mammals takes the form of calcium oscillations.

Calcium ions are released from intracellular storage in the endoplasmic reticulum, free in the cytosol, they are intracellular messengers and act as modulator of the processors in the early steps of fertilization and early development. Mammalian oocytes are activated by intracellular calcium (Ca^{2+}) oscillations following gamete fusion. Recent evidences implicate a sperm specific phospholipase C zeta (PLCζ), which is introduced into the oocyte following membrane fusion, as the responsible factor.[52]

Different methods have been proposed to overcome oocyte activation failure in ICSI cycles, including electrical, mechanical, and chemical oocyte activation. In AOA, sperm oocyte fusion gives rise to intracellular calcium oscillations and are maintained few hours till pronuclei formation.[53,54] Calcium rises after ICSI as a result of artificial calcium influx in the surrounding medium. This increased calcium is extremely important and essential for cytoplasmic and nuclear changes. Assisted oocyte activation is being increasingly applied in human assisted reproduction to restore fertilization and PRs in couples with a history of ICSI fertilization failure. However, controversy still exists mainly because the artificial activating agents do not mimic precisely the initial physiological processes of mammalian oocyte activation, which has led to safety concerns.[55]

Important evidence appeared that the conditions in which activation takes place are very important for the success rate and can vary a lot. Varying concentration of both ionomycin and calcium ions in culture media used during AOA have significant effects on calcium release and further embryonic development potential. The number of children born after AOA is relatively small for statistical analysis. Patients showing compromised fertilization can be treated with artificial oocyte activation which has a great potential in the fertilization rate below 30% in a standard ICSI cycle.[56]

◼ MITOCHONDRIAL DNA LOAD MEASUREMENT

The functional role of mitochondria in infertility is becoming an increasingly important consideration. The mitochondrial deoxyribonucleic acid (mtDNA) in oocytes or embryos have been shown to be involved in some causes of infertility: ovarian insufficiency,[57] endometriosis,[58] female age,[59] and aneuploidy of embryos.[60] Mitochondrial function has also been proposed as a biomarker for embryo implantation.[61]

It is learnt that embryos with elevated mtDNA content have a lower chance to produce an ongoing pregnancy. About one-third to one-quarter of the morphologically and chromosomally normal embryos fail to implant. Research has been focused on new technologies, such as metabolomics,[62] that would assess embryo viability and ultimately allow transfer of a single competent embryo. One important factor in embryo implantation potential could be an adequate energy supply.[63] It has been speculated that both mtDNA heteroplasmy[64] and copy number[59,60,65,66] may contribute to embryo implantation potential. However, conflicting results in this area have already challenged the potential significance of mtDNA in embryo implantation[67,68] and further studies are needed in order to provide clarity.

It has been estimated that metaphase II oocytes contain ~10^5 mtDNA copies, but since no replication of the mtDNA occurs until the blastocyst stage of embryonic development, the mtDNA molecules are divided over the cleaving cells.[59] In 2015, two papers were published reporting an association between higher mtDNA level and lower implantation potential in blastocyst pointing to disturbed energy provision and metabolic stress in embryos with a higher mtDNA content.

Mitochondrial DNA quantification can serve as a biomarker of embryo viability. Elevated mtDNA is accompanied by implantation failure in cases which it was detected.[65] Relative mitochondrial DNA quantity between implanted and nonimplanted embryos was insignificant.[67] Mitochondrial DNA levels were found to be largely equal between blastocysts stratified by ploidy, age or implantation potential.[68]

Currently, there is no evidence that selection through mtDNA load measurement increases LBR. Application of the technique should therefore strictly be limited for research purpose and this should be clearly communicated to the patient.[69]

SPINDLE IMAGING

Oocyte quality is a key limiting factor in female fertility, reflecting the intrinsic developmental potential of an oocyte, and has a crucial role not only in fertilization, but also in subsequent development.[70]

Oocytes exhibiting a meiotic spindle had a significantly higher fertilization rate and a lower rate of abnormal fertilization.[71]

In the first meiotic division because of failure to resolve chiasmata between homologous chromosomes at anaphase I, disturbances in the recombination pathway and premature separation of sister chromatid; error occurs. Nondisjunction of meiotic spindles results in aneuploid gametes and aneuploid embryos. Preincubation between oocyte collection and denudation up to 3 hours after retrieval in ICSI may not increase the percentage of mature oocytes but improves the fertilization and IRs.[72] Oocyte spindle imaging has proven to be an accurate indicator for assessing oocyte maturity.[73] The sperm injection should be achieved without any delay after oocyte denudation to keep good fertilization results. The placement of the sperm during ICSI relative to the presumed location of the meiotic spindle significantly impacts fertilization and high-quality embryo development. Sperm deposition in the M-II spindle area should be avoided. Embryo development is improved by decreasing the distance between the sperm cell and the spindle.[74] Spindle imaging is found to be important tool for predicting ART outcome.[75]

The recent introduction of a new type of polarized light microscope facilitates a noninvasive visualization of the meiotic spindle in the live human oocyte, thereby enabling a better assessment of oocyte meiotic stage **(Figs. 5A and B)**.[75]

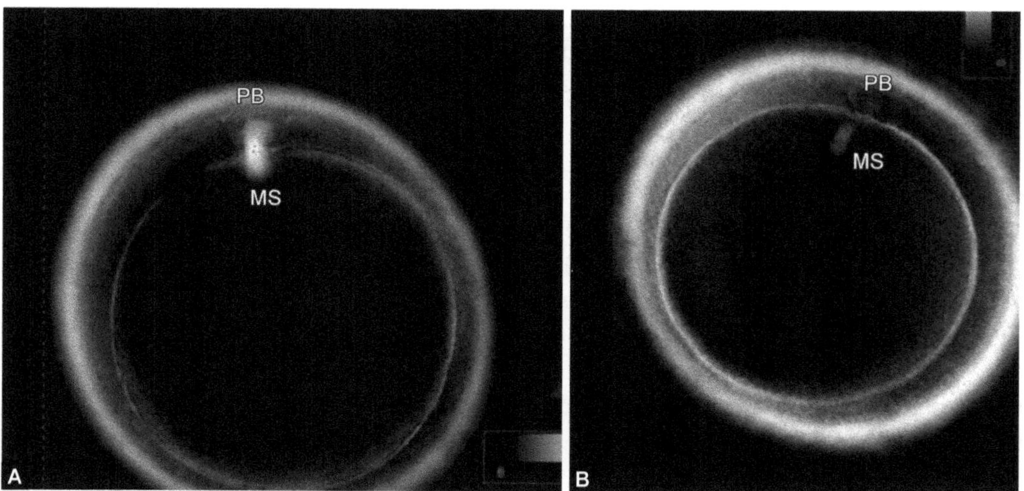

Figs. 5A and B: Assessment of oocyte meiotic stage: (A) Oocyte (with meiotic spindle); (B) Oocyte (in telophase). (MS: meiotic spindle; PB: polar body)

Disruption of the meiotic spindle can lead to rearrangement of chromosomes in the cytoplasm and may contribute to aneuploidy after fertilization.[76] Oocytes at high risk for nondisjunction or oocytes which have failed to fully organize their meiotic spindle and not reached meiotic maturity can be observed by spindle imaging. It suggests that the 11 o'clock position may be the preferred position of the polar body during sperm injection.[76,77] The location of the polar body is only a crude measure for spindle position because these do not always coincide as evidenced by immunostaining. Meiotic spindle imaging can help assess oocytes for quality and select best quality oocytes and also excludes those which do not have meiotic spindle or are in telophase.

Fertilization rates and embryo quality are independent of the position of the meiotic spindle and the polar body.[78] This also is very beneficial for oocyte vitrification where we require to choose oocytes with best reproductive prognosis.

Higher rate of blastocyst formation is seen in MII oocytes with a spindle size of 90–120 um in comparison with the oocytes with spindles outside of that size range suggesting that the measurement of the meiotic spindle size would have positive predictive value for human embryo development potential.[79]

BLASTOCYST CULTURE

Prolonging embryo culture *in vitro* undoubtedly requires greater consistency of laboratory techniques. Increase in its use will depend on increase knowledge of the metabolic requirements of preimplantation embryos and quality control of commercially available culture media. Transfer at blastocyst stage showed increased Live Birth Rates.[80] Advances in understanding the different metabolic needs of cleavage- and blastocyst-stage embryos have resulted in the development of sequential media systems, which have improved the capability of *in vitro* blastocyst formation. Blastocyst culture has higher IRs and LBRs. It has the potential to select the most viable embryos for transfer and also reduce the number of embryos transferred.

Culturing the embryos till cleavage-stage or blastocyst-stage has always been debatable. A committee opinion of ASRM supports blastocyst transfer in good prognosis patients. Elective single embryo transfer should be routinely used to minimize the high risk of multiples in good-prognosis patients.[56] Blastocyst culture has reduced multiple gestations and also increased the IRs. Implantation *in vivo* occurs on Day 5–7 hence culturing till blastocyst stage gives the better synchrony between embryo and endometrium at the time of transfer.[81]

Extended culture has raised obstetric complications and prenatal risks compared to Day 3 cleavage-stage transfer. Blastocyst transfer is associated with higher risk of preterm birth and large for gestational age rates among infants. Despite this blastocyst transfer is also associated with higher delivery rates. Regulatory authorities have recognized their encouragement of single embryo transfer to reduce multiple PRs, still the greatest complication of ART. Embryos which reach the blastocyst stage have been said to be more physiological and thus better able to select themselves for viability.[82]

A recent Cochrane review (Blake et al., 2007) of evidence-based data from RCTs concluded that there is a significant difference in PR and LBR in favor of blastocyst transfer in good prognosis patients, and those with high numbers of 8-cell embryos on Day 3 are the most favored subgroup. No clear recommendation for blastocyst culture and transfer in the general IVF population was given.[29]

Nevertheless, we still believe that blastocyst culture should be used with caution—"as a tool for embryo selection and for enhancing success rates in frozen ART cycles. But we still need to consider whether blastocyst culture should be the gold standard in fresh ART cycles given the adverse risks found in our study", —said by Dr Spangmose.[82] Extended culture allows evaluation of genome activation of the embryo, looking for the embryos that do not reach eight-cell stage hence has lower rates of early abortion.[32]

Only a fraction of cleavage-stage embryos reaches the blastocyst stage, it is currently unknown how many of the other embryos could potentially result in a live birth if transferred at the cleavage-stage. Reproducibility of new information suggests that embryo selection at the eight-cell stage can be as effective as Day 5 transfers, in order to reduce multiple pregnancies while maintaining a high PR.[30]

ASSISTED HATCHING

In case of embryos with thick or dense zona pellucida (ZP), assisted hatching (AH) before transfer is beneficial. Normal embryo hatching is accomplished predominantly by zona lysis and not by pressure exerted by the expanding blastocyst.[31]

A thick ZP may be associated with advanced woman's age or poor embryo quality and *in vitro* culture conditions. ZP is dissolved in lysine, therefore quantitative or qualities deficiencies in its secretion could result in hatching impairment.[83] Advanced maternal age and *in vitro* culture conditions affect the elasticity and thinning of the ZP which are essential for hatching process.

Assisted hatching is a technique wherein a deficiency is made in the ZP either mechanically, chemically or by using LASER. Assisted hatching is proposed to aid in implantation and improve the PRs especially in patients with recurrent implantation failure (RIF).[84]

Assisted hatching has been widely used as an adjunct to standard ART[85] without evidence to support its use and in some cases with a negative consequence.[86-89]

One study aimed to assess the effect of laser-assisted zona hatching technology (LAH) during the frozen-thawed D3 embryos on pregnancy outcomes in patients with previous repeated failures IVF-embryo transfer (IVF-ET). The study showed that LAH via ZP thinning significantly improves clinical outcomes, particularly clinical pregnancy and IRs, associated with FET cycles among patients with previous repeated failure.[90]

LAH is associated with a higher CPR, embryo IR, and multiple PR in women with cryopreserved-thawed embryos. However, LAH is unlikely to increase LBRs and miscarriage rates.

Most studies suggest the hypothesis that AH improves CPR in patients who have had prior failed IVF cycles or poor prognosis. However, there is insufficient evidence that AH improves LBRs in these populations.[79] The American Society of Reproductive Medicine which suggested that individual ART programs should evaluate their own unique patient populations in order to determine which subgroups may benefit from AH.[91]

However, another study says AH cannot currently be recommended as collated results showed no overall benefit to CPRs or live birth rates. There is a significant lack of robust evidence in this field, and areas in particular need of further research have been highlighted.[92]

Assisted hatching increases chance of achieving clinical pregnancy and multiple pregnancy.[93]

The National Institute for Clinical Excellence (NICE) guidelines (2013) state that "assisted hatching is not recommended because it has not been shown to improve PRs".

Assisted hatching through partial zona dissection prior to embryo transfer does not improve pregnancy and embryo IRs in unselected patients undergoing IVF or ICSI.[94] There is good evidence that AH slightly improves CPRs, particularly in poor prognosis patients, including those with prior failed IVF cycles. Due to a limited number of studies, there is insufficient evidence to conclude that AH improves LBRs.[95]

TIME-LAPSE IMAGING

Time-lapse (TL) imaging helps us to continuously monitor the embryo development and morphokinetic parameters based on which embryos can be selected for transfer. Embryo selection becomes an important issue while considering elective single embryo transfer.

Though TL system helps us to study the morphokinetics and several changes occurring in the embryo which can be missed out in routine morphological assessment, few studies are supportive of its use and there is no strong evidence in favor of TL system in improving ART success.

The usefulness of TL imaging in human IVF has been well debated. Among the proposed benefits that have been put forward are "not missing important events during culture", quality control, teaching applications, more information to the patient and, of course, an increase in LBR.

This new technology has been tested as a predictor of blastocyst development, implantation success as well as aneuploidy detection. The use of TL systems may reduce early pregnancy loss, increase eSETs, and limit multiple pregnancies through better embryo selection. However, the quality of the studies and hence the evidence so far, is low-to-moderate quality.[96]

After publication of a series of encouraging retrospective studies, an RCT reported a significantly higher ongoing pregnancy rate (OPR) and IR with the use of embryoscope.[97] Another RCT also found OPR increasing from 40.4% to 68.9% ($p = 0.02$) following TL imaging.[98] No difference in LBRs, CPRs, and miscarriages could be found in a recent Cochrane review of two published RCTs and one study presenting interim analysis.[99] They concluded that there was insufficient evidence to choose between TL imaging and conventional morphological assessment.

Correlation has been found between TL scoring of embryos and blastocyst development in currently available retrospective and few nonrandomized prospective data. The value of morphokinetic assessment in short-listing euploid embryos for transfer has yet to be evaluated in large prospective trials. Until good quality RCT evidence is available TL imaging should be offered only in certain circumstances such as RIF after counseling as to its cost-effectiveness.[100]

Time-lapse imaging is a tool which confers a number of practical benefits to the IVF laboratory. The future challenge for TL imaging is to find the best role in the IVF laboratory and to reduce implementation and consumable costs.[69]

PREIMPLANTATION GENETIC TESTING

Preimplantation genetic testing (PGT) was initially done for couples who were at risk for genetic disorders. Later it was suggested that by applying preimplantation genetic screening (PGS), euploid embryos can be selected for transfer which might improve the ART outcome.[101]

The previous terms of preimplantation genetic diagnosis (PGD) and PGS have been replaced by the term PGT, following a revision of terminology used in infertility care (Zegers-Hochschild et al., 2017). PGT is defined as a test performed to analyze the DNA from oocytes (polar bodies) or embryos (cleavage-stage or blastocyst-stage) for HLA typing or for determining genetic abnormalities. This includes PGT for aneuploidy (PGT-A), PGT for monogenic/single gene defects (PGT-M) and PGT for chromosomal structural rearrangements (PGT-SR) (Zegers-Hochschild et al., 2017). PGT for chromosomal numerical aberrations of high genetic risk are included within PGT-SR in the data collections of the ESHRE PGT consortium.[102] PGT was initially done for couples who were at risk for genetic disorders. Later it was suggested that by applying PGS, euploid embryos can be selected for transfer which might improve the ART outcome.

Extra or missing chromosomes leads to miscarriage or a chromosome syndrome like Down's syndrome which occurs during embryo development and are not related to inherit genetic risks. These chromosomal abnormalities hamper embryo implantation and can be determined by PGT-A whereas heritable genetic mutation that can be passed on to the offspring are detected by PGT-M.

Molecular techniques have been utilized during IVF cycles to determine ploidy including fluorescence *in situ* hybridization (FISH), comparative genomic hybridization (CGH), array CGH (aCGH), digital polymerase chain reaction (dPCR), single-nucleotide polymorphism (SNP) array, real-time quantitative PCR (qPCR), and next-generation sequencing (NGS). These technologies vary in terms of cost and time to completion and few of these methods allow for fresh embryo transfer.[103]

Preimplantation genetic diagnosis and PGS are treatment options that are relatively unregulated and lack standardization compared with other forms of diagnostic testing.[104] Biopsy of blastocyst trophectoderm cells, followed by vitrification of embryos and sample analysis using NGS has become the gold standard method of PGT-A. One of the main reasons for implantation failure and pregnancy loss is the presence of chromosome abnormalities (aneuploidy) in embryonic cells.

Aneuploidy is detrimental to development. The pregenetic testing are capable of determining normal chromosomal embryo, aneuploidy or mixture of normal and abnormal cells (i.e. mosaic) is debatable. To avoid the disadvantages of performing an invasive embryo biopsy with its associated risk and subjecting the preimplantation embryos to an accurate noninvasive method to obtain representative DNA would be ideal for diagnostic PGD/PGS testing in IVF centers.

Hypothesis that blastocysts having unusually high levels of mtDNA detected in the trophectoderm have greatly reduced implantation potential, but there remain significant areas where further validation is necessary and where our understanding is currently inadequate.[105] Clinical outcome in PGT-A is age dependent.[106] PGS cases rather than the

PGD cases showed higher IRs (26.4% vs 20.3%), OPRs (19.5% vs 16.4%), and CPRs (28.6% vs 23.3%). IRs (30.3% vs 23.7%), CPRs (39.2% vs 25.2%), and OPRs (25.7% vs 17.5%) were significant higher in the blastocyst evaluation group than cleavage-stage evaluation group.[107,108] Negative effects on trophectoderm biopsy shows less embryo viability then Day 3 biopsy because trophectoderm biopsy removes only trophectoderm cells, not cells with fetal fate.

Although PGT-A remains controversial in clinical practice, the following indications for its use have been reported: Advanced female/maternal age (AMA), RIF, and recurrent miscarriage (RM). It should be noted that couples with a history of RM have a high chance of successfully conceiving naturally, and in severe male factor.

■ DISCUSSION

Many adjuvants are currently being offered for the couples seeking infertility treatments. The studies on the adjuvants need to be RCTs or placebo studies. However, due to the multitude of factors affecting the outcome of the ART cycles and due to heterogeneity in the studies as well as small sample size, none of the adjuvants have been validated for routine use by any of the regulatory bodies worldwide. N Gleichr, VA Kushnir and DH Barad[104] suggest that random use of the adjuvants have in fact led to the probable decline in the IVF birth rates globally. The authors cite the transition of the IVF centers from being result driven to be modified by industrialization (transition from private practice model to investor-driven industry) and commoditization (primary emphasis on revenue rather than IVF outcomes).

Till date, none of these "add-ons" are considered effective and safe and are not recommended for routine practice by the HFEA©[109] ASRM-SART, ESHRE, NICE, and Australian Fertility Society **(Table 1)**.

Before starting any adjuvant therapy or before applying any new technique, it is the responsibility of the clinician to analyze whether there is any proven advantage of the adjuvant. Also, the risk benefit ratio and the cost benefit ratio have to be taken into account. The effect of the adjuvants on the growth and development of the IVF babies have to be followed up and monitored. Follow-up studies on the physical, neurological, psychological, and sexual development of the babies born out of ART are needed to come to a conclusion.[84]

Infertility experts offering ART treatment naturally want to do the very best they can to improve the chances of pregnancy; the infertile couples too are susceptible to the suggestion that adjuvant therapies will improve that chance. The cost of assisted conception is materially increased by the addition of adjuvants to the extent in some cases that the basic cost may double. Worldwide, treatment costs are often

TABLE 1: HFEA- Traffic light rating system for treatment add-ons in ART.

Add-on test	HFEA rating
Assisted hatching	Amber
AOA	Amber
e-Freeze	Amber
Embryo glue	Amber
PGS (preimplantation genetic screening)	Amber-D5 Red- D3
Time-lapse imaging	Amber
IMSI	Red
pICSI	Red
Sperm DNA fragmentation	No rating given currently

Green: >1 good quality RCT. Procedure is effective and safe. Currently none of the treatment add-ons have been rated green
Amber: Small or conflicting body of evidence, further research still required, technique not recommended for routine use.
Red: No evidence to show that the treatment is effective and safe.
(AOA: artificial oocytes activation; DNA: deoxyribonucleic acid; HFEA: Human Fertilization and Embryology Authority; IMSI: intracytoplasmic morphologically selected sperm injection; PICSI: physiological intracytoplasmic sperm injection)

borne by the patient and the consequence of escalation of costs can be a crippling burden of debt, increased psychological stress and ultimately reduced access to care, most acutely felt in economically challenged situations. Furthermore, the fact that practitioners promulgate adjuvant therapies despite limited or absent evidence, with risks, raises the question of ethical practice.

CONCLUSION

In conclusion, caution should be exercised in prescribing adjuvants in IVF, either individually or in combination as further research is needed to ascertain their efficacy.[92]

REFERENCES

1. European Society of Human Reproduction and Embryology. More than 8 million babies born from IVF since the world's first in 1978: European IVF pregnancy rates now steady at around 36 percent, according to ESHRE monitoring. ScienceDaily; 2018.
2. Duran-Retamal M, Morris G, Achilli C, et al. Live birth and miscarriage rate following intracytoplasmic morphologically selected sperm injection vs intracytoplasmic sperm injection: An updated systematic review and meta-analysis. Acta Obstet Gynecol Scand; 2019. doi: 10.1111/aogs.13703. [Epub ahead of print].
3. Goswami G, Sharma M, Jugga D, et al. Can intracytoplasmic Morphologically Selected Spermatozoa Injection be Used as First Choice of Treatment for Severe Male Factor Infertility Patients? J Hum Reprod Sci. 2018;11:40-4.
4. Oliveira JB, Cavagna M, Petersen CG, et al. Pregnancy outcomes in women with repeated implantation failures after intracytoplasmic morphologically selected sperm injection (IMSI). Reprod Biol Endocrinol. 2011;9:99.
5. De Vos A, Van de Velde H, Bocken G, et al. Does intracytoplasmic morphologically selected sperm injection improve embryo development? A randomized sibling-oocyte study. Hum Reprod. 2013;28(3):617-26.
6. Leandri RD, Gachet A, Pfeffer J, et al. Is intracytoplasmic morphologically selected sperm injection (IMSI) beneficial in the first ART cycle? a multicentric randomized controlled trial. Andrology. 2013;1(5):692-7.
7. Lo Monte G, Murisier F, Piva I, et al. Focus on intracytoplasmic morphologically selected sperm injection (IMSI): a mini-review. Asian J Androl. 2013;15(5):608-15.
8. Knez et al. The IMSI procedure improves poor embryo development in the same infertile couples with poor semen quality: A comparative prospective randomized study. Reproductive Biology and Endocrinology. 2011;9:123.
9. Huszar G, Jakab A, Sakkas D, et al. Fertility testing and ICSI sperm selection by hyaluronic acid binding: clinical and genetic aspects. Reprod Biomed Online. 2007;14:650-63.
10. Avalos-Durán G, Cañedo-Del Ángel AME, Rivero-Murillo J, et al. Physiological ICSI (PICSI) vs. Conventional ICSI in Couples with Male Factor: A Systematic Review. JBRA Assist Reprod. 2018;22(2):139-47.
11. Mokánszki A1, Tóthné EV, Bodnár B, et al. 2014 Aug. Is sperm hyaluronic acid binding ability predictive for clinical success of intracytoplasmic sperm injection: PICSI vs. ICSI?;60(6):348-54. SystBiolReprod Med. doi: 10.3109/19396368.2014.948102.
12. Dyer SJ, Patel M. The economic impact of infertility on women in developing countries—a systematic review. Facts Views Vis Obstet Gynaecol Reprod Health. 2012;4:102-9.
13. Simon L, Murphy K, Shamsi MB, et al. Paternal influence of sperm DNA integrity on early embryonic development. Hum Reprod. 2014;29:2402-12.
14. Worrilow KC, Eid S, Woodhouse D, et al. Use of hyaluronan in the selection of sperm for intracytoplasmic sperm injection (ICSI): significant improvement in clinical outcomes—multicenter, double-blinded and randomized controlled trial. Hum Reprod. 2013;28(2):306-14.
15. Oliva R. Protamines and male infertility. Hum Reprod Update. 2006;12:417-35.
16. Aitken RJ, De Iuliis GN, Finnie JM, et al. Analysis of the relationships between oxidative stress, DNA damage and sperm vitality in a patient population: development of diagnostic criteria. Hum Reprod. 2010;25:2415-26.
17. Zini A. Are sperm chromatin and DNA defects relevant in the clinic? Syst Biol Reprod Med. 2011;57:78-85.
18. Evenson DP, Larson KL, Jost LK. Sperm chromatin structure assay: its clinical use for detecting sperm DNA fragmentation in male infertility and comparisons with other techniques. J Androl. 2002;23:25-43.
19. Spano M, Bonde JP, Hjollund HI, et al. Sperm chromatin damage impairs human fertility. The Danish First Pregnancy Planner Study Team. Fertil Steril. 2000;73:43-50.
20. Simon L, Zini A, Dyachenko A, et al. A systematic review and meta-analysis to determine the effect of sperm DNA damage on in vitro fertilization and intracytoplasmic sperm injection outcome. Asian J Androl. 2017;19:80-90.
21. Bungum M, Humaidan P, Axmon A, et al. Sperm DNA integrity assessment in prediction of assisted reproduction technology outcome. Hum Reprod. 2007;22:174-79.
22. Duran EH, Morshedi M, Taylor S, et al. Sperm DNA quality predicts intrauterine insemination outcome: a prospective cohort study. Hum Reprod. 2002;17:3122-28.
23. Simon L, Liu L, Murphy K, et al. Comparative analysis of three sperm DNA damage assays and sperm nuclear protein content in couples undergoing assisted reproduction treatment. Hum Reprod. 2014;29:904-17.

24. Zhang Z, Zhu L, Jiang H, et al. Sperm DNA fragmentation index and pregnancy outcome after IVF or ICSI: a meta-analysis. J Assist Reprod Genet. 2015;32:17-26.

25. Collins JA, Barnhart KT, Schlegel PN. Do sperm DNA integrity tests predict pregnancy with in vitro fertilization? Fertil Steril. 2008;89:823-31.

26. Wdowiak A, Bakalczuk S, Bakalczuk G. The effect of sperm DNA fragmentation on the dynamics of the embryonic development in intracytoplasmatic sperm injection. Reprod Biol. 2015;15:94-100.

27. Osman A, Alsomait H, Seshadri S, et al. The effect of sperm DNA fragmentation on live birth rate after IVF or ICSI: a systematic review and meta-analysis. Reprod Biomed Online. 2015;30:120-7.

28. Simon L, Emery BR, Carrell DT. Review: diagnosis and impact of sperm DNA alterations in assisted reproduction. Best Pract Res Clin Obstet Gynaecol. 2017;44:38-56.

29. Weissman A, Biran G, Nahum H, et al. Blastocyst culture and transfer: lessons from an unselected, difficult IVF population. Reprod Biomed Online. 2008;17:220-8.

30. Abdelmassih V Balmaceda JP, Nagy ZP, et al. ICSI and day 5 embryo transfers: higher implantation rates and lower rate of multiple pregnancy with prolonged culture. Reprod Biomed Online. 2001;3:216-20.

31. Gordon JW, Dapunt U. A new mouse model for embryos with a hatching deficiency and its use to elucidate the mechanism of blastocyst hatching. Fertil Steril. 1993;59:1296-301.

32. Sepulveda SJ, Portella JR, Noriega LP, et al. Extended culture up to the blastocyst stage: a strategy to avoid multiple pregnancies in assisted reproductive technologies. Biol Res. 2011;44:195-9.

33. Ahmad Majzoub, Ashok Agarwal, Sandro C Esteves. Sperm DNA fragmentation: overcoming standardization obstacles. Transl Androl Urol. 2017;6:S419-21.

34. Zini A, Sigman M. Are tests of sperm DNA damage clinically useful? Pros and cons. J Androl. 2009;30:219-29.

35. Chronopoulou E, Harper JC. IVF culture media: past, present and future. Hum Reprod Update. 2015;21(1):39-55.

36. Siristatidis C, Vogiatzi P, Salamalekis G, et al. Granulocyte macrophage colony stimulating factor supplementation in culture media for subfertile women undergoing assisted reproduction technologies: a systematic review. Int J Endocrinol. 2013;2013:704967.

37. Bontekoe S, Johnson N, Blake D. Adherence compounds in embryo transfer media for assisted reproductive technologies. Cochrane Database Syst Rev. 2014;(2):CD007421.

38. Fancsovits P, Lehner A, Murber A, et al. Effect of hyaluronan-enriched embryo transfer medium on IVF outcome: a prospective randomized clinical trial. Arch Gynecol Obstet. 2015;291:1173-9.

39. Fu W, Yu M, Zhang XJ. Effect of hyaluronic acid-enriched transfer medium on frozen-thawed embryo transfer outcomes. J Obstet Gynaecol Res. 2018;44:747-55.

40. European Society of Human Reproduction and Embryology. First randomised trial shows IVF culture media affect the outcomes of embryos and babies: Fertility experts call for full information on composition of culture media to be made available. ScienceDaily; 2016. [online] Available from https://www.sciencedaily.com/releases/2016/08/160824084356.htm [Last accessed November, 2019].

41. Kleijkers SH, Mantikou E, Slappendel E, et al. Influence of embryo culture medium (G5 and HTF) on pregnancy and perinatal outcome after IVF: a multicentre RCT. Hum Reprod. 2016;31:2219-30.

42. Ziebe S, Loft A, Povlsen BB, et al. A randomised clinical trial to evaluate the effect of granulocyte-macrophage colony-stimulating factor (GM-CSF) in embryo culture medium for in vitro fertilization. Fertil Steril. 2013;99:1600-9.

43. Sunde A, Brison D, Dumoulin J, et al. Time to take human embryo culture seriously. Hum Reprod. 2016;31:2174-82.

44. Vithoulkas A, Levanduski M, Goudas VT, et al. Co-culture of human embryos with autologous cumulus cell clusters and its beneficial impact of secreted growth factors on preimplantation development as compared to standard embryo culture in assisted reproductive technologies (ART). Middle East Fertil Soc J. 2017;22:317-22.

45. Bhadarka HK, Patel NH, Patel NH, et al. Impact of embryo co-culture with cumulus cells on pregnancy and implantation rate in patients undergoing in vitro fertilization using donor oocyte. Indian J Med Res. 2017;146:341-5.

46. Eyheremendy V, Raffo FG, Papayannis M, et al. Beneficial effect of autologous endometrial cell coculture in patients with repeated implantation failure. Fertil Steril. 2010;93:769-73.

47. Spandorfer SD, Barmat L, Navarro J, et al. Autologous endometrial coculture in patients with a previous history of poor quality embryos. J Assist Reprod Genet. 2002;19:309-12.

48. Spandorfer SD, Pascal P, Parks J, et al. Autologous endometrial coculture in patients with IVF failure: outcome of the first 1,030 cases. J Reprod Med. 2004;49:463-7.

49. Le Saint C, Crespo K, Bourdiec A, et al. Autologous endometrial cell co-culture improves human embryo development to high-quality blastocysts: a randomized controlled trial. Reprod Biomed Online. 2019;38:321-9.

50. Fawzy M, Emad M, Mahran A, et al. Artificial oocyte activation with SrCl2 or calcimycin after ICSI improves clinical and embryological outcomes compared with ICSI alone: results of a randomized clinical trial. Hum Reprod. 2018;33:1636-44.

51. Murugesu S, Saso S, Jones BP, et al. Does the use of calcium ionophore during artificial oocyte activation demonstrate an effect on pregnancy rate? A meta-analysis. Fertil Steril. 2017;108:468-82.

52. Kashir J, Heindryckx B, Jones C, et al. Oocyte activation, phospholipase C zeta and human infertility. Hum Reprod Update. 2010;16:690-703.

53. Yanagida K1, Katayose H, Hirata S, et al. Influence of sperm immobilization on onset of Ca^{2+} oscillations after ICSI. Hum Reprod. 2001;16:148-52.

54. Dozortsev D, Rybouchkin A, De Sutter P, et al. Fertilization and early embryology: Human oocyte activation following intracytoplasmic injection: the role of the sperm cell. Hum Reprod. 1995;10:403-7.

55. Vanden Meerschaut F, Nikiforaki D, Heindryckx B, et al. Assisted oocyte activation following ICSI fertilization failure. Reprod Biomed Online. 2014;28:560-71.

56. Markus Montag, Maria Koster, Katrinvan der Ven,et al. The benefit of artificial oocyte activation is dependent on the fertilization rate in a previous treatment cycle. Reproductive BioMedicine Online;Volume 24, Issue 5, May 2012, Pages 521-526. https://doi.org/10.1016/j. rbmo.2012.02.002

57. May-Panloup P, Boucret L, Chao de la Barca JM, et al. Ovarian ageing: the role of mitochondria in oocytes and follicles. Hum Reprod Update. 2016;22:725-43.

58. Xu B, Guo N, Zhang XM, et al. Oocyte quality is decreased in women with minimal or mild endometriosis. Sci Rep. 2015;5:10779.

59. Fragouli E, Spath K, Alfarawati S, et al. Altered levels of mitochondrial DNA are associated with female age, aneuploidy, and provide an independent measure of embryonic implantation potential. PLoS Genet. 2015;11:e1005241.

60. Diez-Juan A, Rubio C, Marin C, et al. Mitochondrial DNA content as a viability score in human euploid embryos: less is better. Fertil Steril. 2015;104:534-41.

61. Seli E. Mitochondrial DNA as a biomarker for in-vitro fertilization outcome. Curr Opin Obstet Gynecol. 2016;28:158-63.

62. Marhuenda-Egea FC, Martínez-Sabater E, Gonsálvez-Alvarez R, et al. A crucial step in assisted reproduction technology: human embryo selection using metabolomic evaluation. Fertil Steril. 2010;94:772-4.

63. Leese HJ. Metabolism of the preimplantation embryo: 40 years on. Reproduction. 2012;143:417-27.

64. Shamsi MB, Govindaraj P, Chawla L, et al. Mitochondrial DNA variations in ova and blastocyst: implications in assisted reproduction. Mitochondrion. 2013;13:96-105.

65. Fragouli E, McCaffrey C, Ravichandran K, et al. Clinical implications of mitochondrial DNA quantification on pregnancy outcomes: a blinded prospective non-selection study. Hum Reprod. 2017;32:2340-7.

66. Ravichandran K, McCaffrey C, Grifo J, et al. Mitochondrial DNA quantification as a tool for embryo viability assessment: retrospective analysis of data from single euploid blastocyst transfers. Hum Reprod. 2017;32:1282-92.

67. Treff NR, Zhan Y, Tao X, et al. Levels of trophectoderm mitochondrial DNA do not predict the reproductive potential of sibling embryos. Hum Reprod. 2017;32:954-62.

68. Victor AR, Brake AJ, Tyndall JC, et al. Accurate quantitation of mitochondrial DNA reveals uniform levels in human blastocysts irrespective of ploidy, age, or implantation potential. Fertil Steril. 2017;107:34-42.e3.

69. Harper J, Jackson E, Sermon K, et al. Adjuncts in the IVF laboratory: where is the evidence for 'add-on' interventions? Hum Reprod. 2017;32:485-91.

70. Gilchrist RB, Lane M, Thompson JG. Oocyte-secreted factors: regulators of cumulus cell function and oocyte quality. Hum Reprod Update. 2008;14:159-77.

71. García-Oro S, Rey MI, Rodríguez M, et al. Predictive value of spindle retardance in embryo implantation rate. J Assist Reprod Genet. 2017;34:617-25.

72. Takeuchi T1, Colombero LT, Neri QV, et al. Does ICSI require acrosomal disruption? An ultrastructural study. Hum Reprod. 2004;19:114-7.

73. Cohen Y, Malcov M, Schwartz T, et al. Spindle imaging: a new marker for optimal timing of ICSI? Human Reproduction, Volume 19, Issue 3, Pages 649–654, https://doi.org/10.1093/humrep/deh113

74. Blake M, Garrisi J, Tomkin G, et al. Sperm deposition site during ICSI affects fertilization and development. Fertil Steril. 2000;73:31-7.

75. C Madaschi, de Souza Bonetti TC, de Almeida Ferreira Braga DP, et al. Spindle imaging: a marker for embryo development and implantation. 90(1):194-8.

76. Hardarson T, Lundin K, Hamberger L. The position of the metaphase II spindle cannot be predicted by the location of the first polar body in the human oocyte. Hum Reprod. 2000;15:1372-6.

77. Cooke S, Tyler JP, Driscoll GL. Meiotic spindle location and identification and its effect on embryonic cleavage plane and early development. Hum Reprod. 2003;18:2397-405.

78. Rienzi L, Ubaldi F, Martinez F, et al. Relationship between meiotic spindle location with regard to the polar body position and oocyte developmental potential after ICSI. Hum Reprod. 2003;18:1289-93.

79. Ko Honjo, Katsuko Kunitake, Natsumi Aramaki, et al. Meiotic spindle size is a strong indicator of human oocyte quality. Reprod Med. Biol. 2018;17:268-74. DOI: 10.1002/rmb2.12100.

80. Siristatidis C, Vogiatzi P, Salamalekis G, et al. Granulocyte macrophage colony stimulating factor supplementation in culture media for subfertile women undergoing assisted reproduction technologies: a systematic review. Int J Endocrinol. 2013;2013:704967.

81. Practice Committee of the American Society for Reproductive Medicine; Practice Committee of the Society for Assisted Reproductive Technology. Blastocyst culture and transfer in clinically assisted reproduction: a committee opinion. Fertil Steril. 2018;110:1246-52.

82. European Society of Human Reproduction and Embryology. Large cohort study confirms small added obstetric risk from transfer of longer developed embryos: Should blastocyst transfer still be encouraged in IVF Clinics? ScienceDaily; 2019. [online] Available from www.sciencedaily.com/releases/2019/06/190624111553.htm [Last accessed November, 2019].

83. Liu HC, Cohen J, Alikani M, et al. Assisted hatching facilitates earlier implantation. Fertil Steril. 1993;60:871-5.

84. Nagarajan G, Thanikachalam P, Kesavan VR, et al. Adjuvants in Assisted Reproductive Technology. Int J Reprod Med Gynecol. 2019;5(2):032-045.

85. Butts SF, Owen C, Mainigi M, et al. Assisted hatching and intracytoplasmic sperm injection are not associated with improved outcomes in assisted reproduction cycles for diminished ovarian reserve: an analysis of cycles in the United States from 2004 to 2011. Fertil Steril. 2014;102:1041-7.

86. Ge HS, Zhou W, Zhang W, et al. Impact of assisted hatching on fresh and frozen-thawed embryo transfer cycles: a prospective, randomized study. Reprod Biomed Online. 2008;16:589-96.

87. Kissin DM, Kawwass JF, Monsour M, et al. National ART Surveillance System (NASS) Group. Assisted hatching: trends and pregnancy outcomes, United States, 2000-10. Fertil Steril. 2014;102:795-801.

88. Nakasuji T, Saito H, Araki R, et al. Validity for assisted hatching on pregnancy rate in assisted reproductive technology: analysis based on results of Japan Assisted Reproductive Technology Registry System 2010. J Obstet Gynaecol Res. 2014;40:1653-60.

89. Elnahas A, Elnahas T, Azmy O, et al. The use of laser assisted hatching of frozen/thawed embryos versus laser assisted hatching of fresh embryos in human intracytoplasmic sperm injection. J Obstet Gynaecol. 2018;38:729.

90. Lu X, Liu Y, Cao X, et al. Laser-assisted hatching and clinical outcomes in frozen-thawed cleavage-embryo transfers of patients with previous repeated failure. Lasers Med Sci. 2019;34:1137-45.

91. Zeng M, Su S, Li L. The effect of laser-assisted hatching on pregnancy outcomes of cryopreserved-thawed embryo transfer: a meta-analysis of randomized controlled trials. Lasers Med Sci. 2018;33:655-66.

92. Kemp A, El-Toukhy T. A narrative review of adjuvants in in vitro fertilisation: evidence for good clinical practice. J Obstet Gynaecol. 2019;29:1-8.

93. Li D, Yang DL, An J, et al. Effect of assisted hatching on pregnancy outcomes: a systematic review and meta-analysis of randomized controlled trials. Sci Rep. 2016;6:31228.

94. Hellebaut S, De Sutter P, Dozortsev D, et al. Does assisted hatching improve implantation rates after in vitro fertilization or intracytoplasmic sperm injection in all patients? A prospective randomized study. J Assist Reprod Genet. 1996;13:19-22.

95. Practice Committee of the American Society for Reproductive Medicine; Practice Committee of the Society for Assisted Reproductive Technology. Role of assisted hatching in in vitro fertilization: a guideline. Fertil Steril. 2014;102:348-51.

96. Bhide P, Maheshwari A, Cutting R, et al. Time lapse imaging: is it time to incorporate this technology into routine clinical practice? Hum Fertil (Camb). 2017;20:74-9.

97. Rubio I, Galán A, Larreategui Z, et al. Clinical validation of embryo culture and selection by morphokinetic analysis: a

randomized, controlled trial of the EmbryoScope. Fertil Steril. 2014;102:1287-94.e5.

98. Yang Z, Zhang J, Salem SA, et al. Selection of competent blastocysts for transfer by combining time-lapse monitoring and array CGH testing for patients undergoing preimplantation genetic screening: a prospective study with sibling oocytes. BMC Med Genomics. 2014;7:38.

99. Armstrong S, Arroll N, Cree LM, et al. Time-lapse systems for embryo incubation and assessment in assisted reproduction (Review). Cochrane Database Syst Rev. 2015;27:CD011320.

100. Datta AK, Campbell S, Deval B, et al Add-ons in IVF programme—Hype or Hope? Facts Views Vis Obgyn. 2015;7:241-50.

101. Thornhill AR, deDie-Smulders CE, Geraedts JP, et al. ESHRE PGD Consortium 'Best practice guidelines for clinical preimplantation genetic diagnosis (PGD) and Preimplantation genetic screening (PGS)'. Hum Reprod. 2005;20:35-48.

102. PGT Consortium Steering committee, Carvalho F, Coonen E, et al. ESHRE PGT Consortium good practice recommendations for the organisation of preimplantation genetic testing. ESHRE: Belgium; 2017.

103. Practice Committees of the American Society for Reproductive Medicine and the Society for Assisted Reproductive Technology. The use of preimplantation genetic testing for aneuploidy (PGT-A): a committee opinion. Fertil Steril. 2018;109:429-36.

104. Gleicher N, Kushnir VA, Barad DH. Worldwide decline of IVF birth rates and its probable causes. Hum Reprod Open. 2019;2019(3):hoz017.

105. Wells D. Mitochondrial DNA quantity as a biomarker for blastocyst implantation potential. Fertil Steril. 2017;108:742-7.

106. Murphy LA, Seidler EA, Vaughan DA, et al. To test or not to test? A framework for counselling patients on preimplantation genetic testing for aneuploidy (PGT-A). Hum Reprod. 2019;34:268-75.

107. Won SY, Kim H, Lee WS, et al. Pre-implantation genetic diagnosis and pre-implantation genetic screening: two years experience at a single center. Obstet Gynecol Sci. 2018;61:95-101.

108. Kuznyetsov V, Madjunkova S, Antes R, et al. Evaluation of a novel non-invasive preimplantation genetic screening approach. PLoS One. 2018;13:e0197262.

109. hfea.gov.uk

Adjuvants in Male Subfertility

Ameet S Patki, Teena Trivedi Desai

■ INTRODUCTION

The inability to conceive a child is a distressing reality for a large number of couples worldwide in today's era. Male factor alone is responsible for 40% cases of infertility, female factor accounts for 40% of infertility, and in 20% cases combined male and female factors are responsible for infertility. Continuous attempts have been going on since the 19th century to understand the causes of male subfertility. Despite the advances made in the field of infertility, the causes of male subfertility still elude the scientists. Empiric therapies are being used for various forms of male subfertility.[1] Various adjuvant therapies like antioxidants, clomiphene citrate, aromatase inhibitors, human chorionic gonadotropin (hCG), recombinant follicle-stimulating hormone (FSH), growth hormone (GH), and varicocelectomy have been used since a long time.

There has been a lot of emphasis on the use of antioxidants in the management of male subfertility. Oxidative stress occurs when reactive oxygen species (ROS) are in abundance. When ROS is present in high levels in the seminal fluid, they can damage the sperms by altering membrane integrity, affecting sperm motility, morphology and thereby causing sperm cell death.[2] Antioxidants are compounds that reduce or terminate oxidative stress. Oral antioxidants have been used alone or in combination with other agents. Antioxidants are of two types:

1. *Catalytic antioxidants* that activate certain metabolic reactions that interfere with ROS formation and protect against the toxic effects of ROS.
2. *Scavenging antioxidants* that directly react with the oxidant molecules and neutralize them.

■ ANTIOXIDANT THERAPY

Catalytic Antioxidants

N-acetyl Cysteine

It is a sulfhydryl compound, a nontoxic derivative of amino acid L-cysteine. It neutralizes hydrogen peroxide, hypochlorous acid, and hydroxyl radicle and enhances the production of glutathione. It has been found to play an important role in germ cell survival in seminiferous tubules *in vitro*.[3] A randomized controlled trial (RCT) has shown that therapy with N-acetyl cysteine 600 mg daily for 3 months given to men with idiopathic infertility leads to increase in semen volume and sperm motility, and reduces semen viscosity.[4] The preferred dose is 200–500 mg up to three times a day. No significant side-effects have been reported except diarrhea.

Vitamin E

Vitamin E is an important lipid soluble antioxidant molecule in the cell membrane. Alpha tocopherol, the most common and most active form of vitamin E is thought to interrupt lipid peroxidation and enhance the activity of various antioxidants that scavenge free radicles.[5,6] *In vitro* studies suggest that it may enhance sperm motility and improve sperm performance in animals.[7] According to RCT, a dose of 100 mg/ day for 6 months is effective in treating males with oxidative stress.[8-10] Larger doses may interfere with blood clotting factors especially in patients taking anticoagulants.[11] It may be added to cryoprotectants to protect sperms from oxidative stress during cryopreservation and thawing.[12]

Coenzyme Q

Coenzyme Q is a fat soluble substance. There are 10 forms of coenzyme Q and coenzyme Q10 (Ubiquinone) is synthesized by human body. Coenzyme Q10 is found in the sperm-midpiece. It helps in recycling vitamin E and control its pro oxidant capacity and is involved in energy production.[13] Oral dose of 60 mg has been shown to improve fertilization rates without affecting semen parameters and also shown to inhibit hydrogen peroxide formation in seminal fluid.[14,15] Normal dietary intake is 3–6 mg, most of which is derived from meat. A daily therapeutic dose of 3,600 mg is well tolerated by healthy and unhealthy men. Gastrointestinal symptoms have been reported with very high doses.

Carnitine

Carnitine is a small water soluble quaternary ammonium compound. About 75% of which is derived from diet and 25% synthesized from lysine and methionine in kidneys and liver. It is crucial for energy production at mitochondrial level. One study showed that a single dose increases the serum levels of antioxidant enzymes like catalase, superoxide dismutase, and glutathione peroxidase and hence, increased the total antioxidant capacity level.[16] It has a role in sperm energy metabolism and provides primary fuel for sperm motility. Patients with defective sperm motility have been found to have low levels of L-acetyl carnitine/L-carnitine ratio.[17] In a systemic review by Ross et al., oral carnitine has improved sperm motility and concentration.[10,18,19] In addition to this it also protects the sperm DNA and cell membrane from ROS-induced damage and apoptosis.[20-23] A dose of 1–4 g/day can be given. No major side effects except mild gastrointestinal symptoms have been reported. In a randomized controlled trial a daily dose of 2 g, carnitine showed improvement in sperm motility.[20,22] No further improvement is seen after a treatment period of 3–6 months as per all the studies.

Selenium

It is a trace metal found in small amounts in specific proteins called selenoproteins, which help maintain sperm structure integrity. It may protect against oxidative sperm DNA damage and play a role in normal testicular development, spermatogenesis, sperm motility, and function.[24] The exact mechanism of action is not known but it is thought to mediate its antioxidant actions by selenoenzymes like hydroperoxide glutathione peroxidase and sperm capsular selenoproteins.[25-27] It also potentiates the antioxidant action of vitamin E. RCT by Moslemi et al. showed that selenium 200 µg and vitamin E 400 IU given to men with idiopathic asthenospermia for 100 days improved sperm motility and morphology and thus improved spontaneous pregnancy rates.[28] Optimum daily allowance is 200 µg and the maximum dose is 400 µg. Excessive bleeding, hepatorenal dysfunction, hair loss, and brittle nails have been reported with higher doses (>850 µg).[29]

Zinc

Zinc deficiency is associated with abnormal flagella, axonemal disruption, and partial defects of inner dynein arms of microtubular doublets with distorted inner axonemal structure and a poorly formed or absent midpiece of the sperm.[30] RCT by Al Bader et al. and Omu et al.[31] has shown that daily supplementation of 200 mg of zinc for 3 months has reduced the level of tumor necrosis factor, apoptotic factors, antisperm antibodies and DNA fragmentation in seminal fluid and increased the expression and activity of cytokine interleukin 4. The optimum daily allowance of zinc is 15–35 mg/day. High doses have caused breakage of sperm DNA strand in salmon.[32] Use of high dose (150 mg) for prolonged periods leads to toxicity characterized by symptoms such as gastrointestinal symptoms, immune dysfunction, dizziness, anemia, and hypoglycemia in diabetic men.[33]

Pentoxifylline

It is a competitive nonselective phosphodiesterase inhibitor that raises intracellular cAMP levels and reduces inflammation by inhibiting TNF-α and leukotriene synthesis. Studies have shown that supplementation with pentoxifylline reduces ROS production and preserve sperm motility in vitro and improved sperm parameters in vivo.[34-37] Recommended oral dose is 400 mg thrice a day. Nausea, vomiting, dizziness, diarrhea, headache, and tremors have been reported with high doses.

Scavenging Antioxidants

Vitamin C

It is a water soluble vitamin not synthesized by human body. The concentration of vitamin C is 10-fold higher in seminal plasma than serum.[38,39] A dose of 1,000 mg/L has shown to improve sperm viability and motility.[38] At higher doses the pro-oxidant effect may be lost, reducing sperm motility.[40] Studies have documented a reduction in sperm DNA fragmentation with combined supplementation of vitamin C and vitamin E.[41] Another RCT failed to show improvement in semen parameters and pregnancy rate in couples with male factor infertility after administration of vitamin C and vitamin E in doses for 56 days.[42] More studies are required to confirm whether vitamin C supplementation will be effective in patients with sperm DNA damage. Optimum daily allowance is 250–1,000 mg/day. Doses higher than 2,000 mg/day may cause diarrhea, interference in absorption of vitamin B_{12} and copper.

Lycopene

It is a carotenoid compound found in high concentrations in testis and seminal plasma. Lower levels are found in infertile men. One study has shown statistically significant improvement in sperm concentration and motility after administration of 200 mg lycopene twice a day for 3 months.[43] But these effects were seen only in patients with baseline sperm concentration of more than 5 million/mL. Further randomized studies are required to establish the indications of lycopene treatment in male subfertility. Oral dose of 20–30 mg/day can be given.

The evidence for the potential benefits of antioxidant therapy in male subfertility is still uncertain. A Cochrane review in 2011, analyzing 34 RCTs involving 2,876 couples aimed at evaluating the effect of antioxidants in male partners of couples undergoing assisted reproductive techniques.[44] Findings suggest an increase in pregnancy and live birth rates with use of antioxidants. It did not substantiate improvement in semen parameters. Also, it did not conclude that any one antioxidant is better than the other in terms of pregnancy rate or semen parameters. It is also suggested that antioxidants may be beneficial for embryo development by reducing apoptosis. Since male subfertility is multifactorial, definitive conclusion cannot be drawn on the basis of heterogeneous studies on the use of antioxidants in male subfertility.

■ FOLLICLE-STIMULATING HORMONE

As per a study pure FSH, given to men with severe oligoasthenoteratospermia, has improved sperm motility and spontaneous pregnancy rates and pregnancy rates after IVF.[45] RCT, showed that treatment with recombinant FSH, in a dose of 150 IU subcutaneously 3 times a week for 3 months before ICSI, causes improvement in sperm concentration, pregnancy rate, implantation rate, and decreased early pregnancy loss in men with idiopathic oligospermia.[46]

■ GROWTH HORMONE

Growth hormone is expressed in a variety of tissues including testis and exerts an autocrine and paracrine effect on spermatogenesis in male partners with hypogonadotropic hypogonadism who do not respond to gonadotropin or pulsatile luteinizing hormone (LH) therapy.[47] It acts directly and indirectly at the testicular level in the process of spermatogenesis. An open label, nonrandomized controlled study on 14 Indian men between 26 years and 35 years with idiopathic oligoasthenospermia, showed an improvement in semen volume, sperm count, and motility with daily administration of 1.5 IU of growth hormone for 6 months.[48] More studies are required to substantiate the use of GH in cases of male subfertility. Watch for metabolic side-effects when administering growth hormone therapy.

■ HUMAN CHORIONIC GONADOTROPIN

Human chorionic gonadotropin is an LH analog that stimulates Leydig cells in the testis and increases intratesticular and serum levels of testosterone, thereby improving spermatogenesis. It can be given by intramuscular or subcutaneous route. hCG alone has shown to improve semen parameters only for a short duration. A study by Depenbusch et al. has shown that benefits of hCG monotherapy reduce after 12 months of treatment.[49] A recent case series on 49 men with severe oligospermia and azoospermia who had received testosterone therapy were given alternate day 1,500 IU of hCG with other supplement therapy like clomiphene citrate, anastrozole, tamoxifen or recombinant FSH for a period of 14 months showed an improvement in sperm count in 95% cases and achieving a pregnancy with no documented adverse effects.[50] hCG therapy is an effective but underutilized treatment in male subfertility due to the invasive nature of treatment and expense of the drug.

■ CLOMIPHENE CITRATE

It is a selective estrogen receptor modulator (SERM) that blocks the negative feedback mechanism at the level of hypothalamus and pituitary. This increases the levels of FSH and LH and thus increases testosterone levels and improves spermatogenesis.[51] It is not FDA approved for use in men. It has two isoforms–enclomiphene and zuclomiphene. Since it increases FSH levels, it is not useful in men with high FSH levels or those who lack a post treatment FSH surge. This therapy may be considered in patients with idiopathic infertility with a sperm concentration between 10 and 20 million/mL and normal to slightly below normal sperm motility and morphology and low FSH and LH.[52] Some studies have shown an improvement in sperm concentration and pregnancy rates, while some have not shown the same benefits.[51-53] It can be administered in dose of 12.5–400 mg/day. Many dosing regimens have been described like starting 25–50 mg on alternate and increasing to 50 mg daily or giving 100 mg daily. Enclomiphene, one of the isomers of clomiphene citrate has shown to improve morning levels of FSH, LH, testosterone, and estrogen while preserving spermatogenesis as per one study. It is a pure estrogen antagonist as compared to clomiphene which is an agonist and antagonist.[54] It is mostly well tolerated by patients, though gastrointestinal distress, hair loss, and gynecomastia have been reported. Preliminary data on enclomiphene is promising, but more randomized studies and FDA approval are required to substantiate its use as an adjuvant in male subfertility.

AROMATASE INHIBITORS

Aromatase is a cytochrome p450 enzyme found in brain, bone, testis, and prostate of men. It converts testosterone to androstenedione to estradiol and estrone. Estradiol has a negative feedback on hypothalamus and reduces pituitary gonadotropins and hence affects spermatogenesis. Aromatase inhibitors like letrozole and anastrozole inhibit the cytochrome p450 enzyme and prevent the negative feedback of estrogen and hence, lead to stronger gonadotropin releasing hormone (GnRH) pulses and increase FSH levels and spermatogenesis.[51,55,56] They increase testosterone levels without impacting estrogen levels, unlike clomiphene. Letrozole is more potent than anastrozole. A study on men with low testosterone and T/E ratio treated with letrozole has shown increase in serum testosterone, sperm concentration, motility and morphology, and reduced estrogen levels. It can be considered in men with nonobstructive infertility. In the same study about 5% cases female partners of oligospermic men achieved pregnancy and about 4% azoospermic men demonstrated sperms in repeat semen analysis.[55,56] Letrozole can be given in the dose of 2.5 mg once a week to thrice a week. Side effects like headache, deranged liver enzymes and decreased libido have been reported. More RCTs are required to define their role in male subfertility.

THYROID HORMONES

Infertile men with hyperthyroidism have reported with symptoms of decreased libido, erectile dysfunction, premature ejaculation, and signs of hyperestrogenemia like gynecomastia. Sertoli cells of testis express thyroid hormone receptors and the hormone also influences Leydig cells and spermatogenesis. Hyperthyroid and hypothyroid men have shown a lower level of morphologically normal sperms.[57-59] Studies have demonstrated that hyperthyroid men have deranged semen parameters like sperm motility, which can be corrected after treatment of hyperthyroidism.[60] The effect of hypothyroidism on male subfertility is not substantial. A study has shown that hypothyroidism is associated with decreased libido, erectile dysfunction, and abnormal semen parameters like reduced count, motility, and morphology.[61,62] Routine testing for thyroid dysfunction is not recommended as per studies due to low yield and hence, it should not be considered as the sole cause of male subfertility.[63]

PROLACTIN

The role of prolactin in male health is still unknown, though it has been shown that Leydig, Sertoli, and germ cells in testis express prolactin receptors. It can affect spermatogenesis by modulating the LH receptors or activity of spermatogenic enzymes.[64,65] There is conflicting data on the effects of hyperprolactinemia on semen parameters and hence its role in male subfertility is inconclusive.[66]

OBESITY IN MALES

Obesity is on a rise in this day and age. Subfertility and poor sperm parameters are found in obese men.[67] This association may be due to reduced testosterone and sex hormone binding globulin (SHBG) and increased estrogen, body temperature and oxidative stress. The data is conflicting since some studies have found obesity to affect sperm motility and morphology, while others have not.[68-70] One study was able to demonstrate the benefits of sleeve gastrectomy on sperm concentration in oligospermic and azoospermic men.[71]

VARICOCELECTOMY

About 35% of subfertile men have a clinically identifiable varicocele.[72] The suggested mechanism contributing to subfertility is associated with the increased oxidative stress, hormonal imbalance, increase in scrotal temperature, reflux of renal and adrenal metabolites, and testicular hypoperfusion.[73] Studies have shown that varicocelectomy is associated with increased serum testosterone levels.[74] There is evidence to support that varicocelectomy improves outcomes in subfertile males with clinically palpable varicocele.[75] But this improvement is not universally observed in all the men subjected to a surgery. Hence, adjuvant medical therapy after surgery is an option in such patients.

REFERENCES

1. Ko EY, Siddiqi K, Brannigan RE, et al. Empirical medical therapy for idiopathic male infertility: a survey of the American Urological Association. J Urol. 2012;187(3):973-8.
2. Aitken RJ. Free radicles, lipid peroxidation and sperm function. Reprod Fertil Dev. 1995;7(4):659-68.
3. Erkkila K, Hirvonen V, Woukko E, et al. N-acetyl-L-cysteine inhibits apoptosis in human germ cells in vitro. J Clin Endocrinol Metab. 1998;83(7):2523-31.

4. Cifti H, Verit A, Savas M, et al. Effects of N acetyl cysteine for improving semen parameters and oxidative/antioxidant status. Urology. 2009;74:73-6.

5. Ehrenkranz RA. Vit E and the neonate. Am J Dis Child. 1980;134:1157-66.

6. Palamanda JR, Kehrer JP. Involvement of Vit E and protein thiols in inhibition of microsomal lipid peroxidation by glutathione. Lipids. 1993;28:427-31.

7. de Lamirande E, Gangon C. Reactive oxygen species and human spermatozoa II. Depletion of adenosine triphosphate plays an important role in the inhibition of sperm motility. J Androl. 1992;13(5):379-86.

8. Kessopoulou E, Powers HJ, Sharma KK, et al. A double blind randomized placebo cross over controlled trial using antioxidant Vit E to treat reactive oxygen species associated male infertility. Fertil Steril. 1995;64:825-31.

9. Suleiman SA, AliME, Zaki ZM, et al. Lipid peroxidation and human sperm motility: protective role of Vit E. J Androl. 1996;17:530-7.

10. Ross C, Morris Khairy M, et al. A systemic review of the effect of oral antioxidants on male infertility. Reprod Biomed Online. 2010;20:711-23.

11. Steiner M. Influence of Vit E on platelet function in humans. J Am Coll Nutr. 1991;10:466-73.

12. Lewin A, Lavon H. The effect of Coenzyme Q10 on sperm motility and function. Mol Aspects Med. 1997;18(Suppl);S213-9.

13. Thomas SR, Neuzil J, Stocker R. Inhibition of LDL oxidation by ubiquinol-10.A protective mechanism for coenzyme Q in atherogenesis? Mol Aspects Med. 1997:18(Suppl):S85-103.

14. Alleva R, ScararmucciA, Mantero F, et al. The protective role of ubiquinol-10 against formation of lipid hydroperoxidases in human seminal fluid. Mol Aspects Med. 1997:18(Suppl):S221-8.

15. Cao Y, Qu HJ Li P, et al. Single dose administration of L-carnitine improves antioxidant activities in healthy subjects. Tohoku J Exp Med. 2011:224:209-13.

16. Bartellini M, Canale D, Izzo PL, et al. L-carnitine and acetylcarnitine in human sperm with normal and reduced motility. Acta Eur Fertil. 1987:18:29-31.

17. Menchini–Fabris GF, Canale D, Izzo PL, et al. Free L-carnitine in human semen: its variability in different androgenic pathologies. Fertil Steril. 1984;42:263-7.

18. Bornman MS, du Toit D, Otto B et al. Seminal Carnitine, epididymal function and spermatozoal motility. S Afr Med J. 1989;75:20-1.

19. Lenzi A, Lombardo F, Sgro P, et al. Use of carnitine therapy in selected cases of male factor infertility: a double blinded cross-over trial. Fertil Steril. 2003;79:292-300.

20. Arduini A. Carnitine and its acyl esters as secondary antioxidants. Am Heart J. 1992:123:1726-7.

21. Lenzi A, Sgro P, Salacone P, et al. A placebo-controlled double-blinded randomized trial of the use of combined L-carnitine and L-acetyl-carnitine treatment in men with asthenozoospermia. Fertil Steril. 2004;81:1578-84.

22. Cavallini G, Ferraretti AP, GianaroliL, et al. Cinnoxicam and L-carnitine/L-acetyl carnitine treatment for idiopathic and varicocele associated oligoasthenospermia. J Androl. 2004;25:761-70, discussion 71-2.

23. Ursini F, Heim S, Keiss M, et al. Dual function of selenoprotein PHGPx during sperm maturation. Science. 1999;285:1393-6.

24. Roveri A, Casasco A, Maiorino M, et al. Phospholipid hydroperoxide glutathione peroxidase of rat testis. Gonadotropin dependence and immunocytochemical identification. J Biol Chem. 1992;267:6142-6.

25. Alvarez JG, Storey BT. Lipid peroxidation and reactions of superoxide and hydrogen peroxide in mouse spermatozoa. Biol Reprod. 1984;30:833-41.

26. Surai PF, Bleisbois E, Grasseau I, et al. Fatty acid composition ,glutathione peroxidase and superoxide dismutase activity and total antioxidant activity of avian semen. Comp Biochem Physiol B Biochem Mol Biol. 1998;120:527-33.

27. Moslemi MK, Tavanbakshsh S. Selenium-vitamin E supplementation in infertile men: Effect on semen parameters and pregnancy rate. Int J Gen Med. 2011;4:99-104.

28. Yang GQ, Wang SZ, Zouh RH, Sun ZS. Endemic selenium intoxication in humans in China. Am J Clin Nutr. 1983;37:872-81.

29. Omu AE, Al-Azemi MK, Kehinde EO, et al. Indications of the mechanisms involved in improved sperm parameters by zinc therapy. Med Princ Pract. 2008;17:108-16.

30. Al-Bader A, Omu AE, Dashti H. Chronic cadmium toxicity to sperms of heavy cigarette smokers: immunomodulation by zinc. Arch Androl. 1999;43:135-40.

31. Loyd DR, Carmichael PL, Phillip DH. Comparison of formation of 8-hydroxy-2'deoxyguanosine and single and double stranded breaks in DNA mediated by fenton reaction. Chem Res Toxicol. 1998;11:420-7.

32. Porea TJ, Belmont JW, Mahoney DH Jr. Zinc induced anemia and neutropenia in adolescent. J Pediatr. 2000;136:688-90.

33. Gavella M, Lipovac V. Pentoxifylline-mediated reduction of superoxide anion production by human spermatozoa. Andrologia. 1992;24;37-9.

34. Gavella M, Lipovac V, Marotti T. Effect of pentoxifylline on superoxide anion production by human sperm. Int J Androl. 1991;14:320-7.

35. Marrama P, Baraghini GF, Carani C, et al. Further studies on the effect of pentoxifylline on sperm count and motility in patients with idiopathic oligo-astheno-zoospermia. Andrologia. 1985;17:612-6.

36. Yovich JM, Edirisinghe WR, Cummins JM, et al. Influence of pentoxifylline in severe male factor infertility. Fertil Steril. 1990;53:715-22.

37. Dawson EB, Harris WA, Rankin WE, et al. Effect of ascorbic acid on male fertility. Ann N J Acad Sci. 1987;498:312-23.

38. Jacob RA, Pianalto FS, Agee RE. Cellular ascorbate depletion in healthy men. J Nutr. 1992;122:1111-8.

39. Abel BJ, Carswell G, Elton R, et al. Randomised trial of clomiphene citrate treatment and vitamin C for male infertility. Br J Urol. 1982;54:780-4.

40. Greco E, Lacobelli M, Reinzi L, et al. Reduction of incidence of sperm DNA fragmentation by oral antioxidant treatment. J Androl. 2005;26:349-53.

41. Rolf C, Cooper TG, Yeung CH, et al. Antioxidant treatment of patients with asthenozoospermia or moderate oligoasthenozoospermia with high dose vitamin C and vitamin E:a randomised placebo-controlled, double blind study. Hum Reprod. 1999;14:1028-33.

42. Gupta NP, Kumar R. Lycopene therapy in idiopathic male infertility-a preliminary report. Int Urol Nephrol. 2002;34:369-72.

43. Showell MG, Brown J, Yazdani A, et al. Antioxidants for male subfertility. Cochrane Database Syst Rev. 2011;(1):CD007411.

44. Dirnfeld M, Katz G, Calderon I,, et al. Pure follicle stimulating hormone as an adjuvant therapy for selected cases in male infertility during in-vitro fertilization is beneficial. Eur J Obstet Gynecol Reprod Biol. 2000;93(1):105-8.

45. Farrag A, Sagnella F, Pappalardo S, et al. The use of r-FSH in treatment of idiopathic male factor infertility before ICSI. Eur Rev Med Pharmacol Sci. 2015;19(12):2162-67.

46. Magon N, Singh S, et al. Growth hormone in male infertility. Indian J Endo Metab. 2011;15(Supp 3):S248-9.

47. Kalra S, Kalra B, Sharma A. Growth hormone improves semen volume, sperm count and motility in men with idiopathic normogonadotropic infertility. Endocr Abstr. 2008;16:P613.

48. Depenbusch M, von Eckardstein S, Simoni M, et al. Maintenance of spermatogenesis in hypogonadotropic hypogonadal men with human chorionic gonadotropin alone. Eur J Endocrinol. 2002;147:617-24.

49. Wenker EP, Dupree JM, Langille GM, et al. The use of HCG-based combination therapy for recovery of spermatogenesis after testosterone use. J Sex Med. 2015;12:1334-7.

50. Chenab M, Madala A, Trussell JC. On-label and off-label drugs used in the treatment of male infertility. Fertil Steril. 2015;103(3):595-604.

51. Bridges N, Trofimenko V, Fields S, et al. Male factor infertility and clomiphene citrate: a meta-analysis: The effect of clomiphene citrate on oligospermia. Urol Pract. 2015;2:199-205.

52. Chua ME, Escusa KG, Luna S, et al. Revisiting oestrogen antagonists(clomiphene and tamoxifen) as medical empiric therapy for idiopathic male infertility: a meta-analysis. Andrology. 2013;1:749-57.

53. Wiehle RD, Fontenot GK, Wike J, et al. Enclomiphene citrate stimulates testosterone production while preventing oligospermia: a randomised phase II clinical trial comparing topical testosterone. Fertil Steril. 2014;102:720-7.

54. Schlegel PN. Aromatase inhibitors for male infertility. Fertil Steril. 2012;98:1359-62.

55. Stephens SM, Polotsky AJ. Big enough for an aromatase inhibitor? How adiposity affects male infertility. Semen Reprod Med. 2012;31:251-7.

56. Mintziori G, Kita M, Duntas L, et al. Consequences of hyperthyroidism in male and female infertility: pathophysiology and current management. J Endocrinol Invest. 2016;39:849-53.

57. Krassas GE, Pontikides N. Male reproductive function in relation with thyroid alterations. Best Pract Res Clin Endocrinol Metab. 2004;18:183-95.

58. Kumar A, Shekhar S, Dhole B. Thyroid and male reproduction. Indian J Endocrinol Metab. 2014;18:23-31.

59. Krassas GE, Pontides N, Deligianni V, et al. A prospective controlled study of the impact of hyperthyroidism on reproductive function in males. J Clin Endocrinol Metab. 2002;87:3667-71.

60. Nikoobakht MR, Aloosh M, Nikoobakht N, et al. The role of hypothyroidism in male infertility and erectile dysfunction. Urol J. 2012;9:405-9.

61. Poppe K, Glinoer D, Tournaye H, et al. Is systematic screening for thyroid disorders indicated in subfertile men? Eur J Endocrinol. 2006;154:363-6.

62. Lotte F, Maseroli E, Fralassi N, et al. Is thyroid hormone evaluation of clinical value in the work-up of males of infertile couples? Hum Reprod. 2016;31:518-29.

63. Binart N, Melaine N, Pineau C, et al. Male reproductive function is not affected in prolactin receptor-deficient mice. Endocrinology. 2003;144:3779-82.

64. Mancini A, Guitelman A, Levallo O, et al. Bromocriptine in the management of infertile men after surgery of prolactin secreting adenomas. J Androl. 1984;5:294-6.

65. Okada H, Iwamoto T, Fujioka H, et al. Hyperprolactinaemia among infertile patients and its effect on sperm functions. Andrologia. 1996;28:197-202.

66. Raad G, Hazzouri M, Bottini S, et al. Paternal obesity: how bad is it for sperm quality and progeny health? Basic Clin Androl. 2017;27:20.

67. Hammoud AO, Gibson M, Peterson CM, et al. Impact of male obesity on infertility: a critical review of current literature. Fertil Steril. 2008;90:897-904.

68. Jensen TK, Andersson AM, Jørgensen N, et al. Body mass index in relation to semen quality and reproductive hormones among 1558 Danish men. Fertil Steril. 2004;82:863-70.

69. Kort HI, Massey JB, Elsner CW, et al. Impact of body mass index on sperm quantity and quality. J Androl. 2006;27:450-2.

70. El Bardisi H, Majzoub A, Arafa M, et al. Effect of bariatric surgery on semen parameters and sex hormone concentrations: a prospective study. Reprod Biomed Online. 2016;33:606-11.

71. Gorelick JI, Goldstein M. Loss of fertility in men with varicocele. Fertil Steril. 1993;59:613-6.

72. Hamada A, Esteves SC, Agarwal A, et al. Insight into oxidative stress in varicocele associated male infertility: part 2. Nat Urol. 2013:10;26-37.

73. Zohdy W, Ghazi S, Arafa M. Impact of varicocelectomy on gonadal and erectile functions in men with hypogonadism and infertility. J Sex Med. 2011;8:885-93.

74. Practice Committee of the American Society for Reproductive Medicine; Society for Male Reproduction and Urology. Report on varicocele and infertility: a committee opinion. Fertil Steril. 2014;102:1556-60.

75. Garg H, Kumar R. Empirical drug therapy for idiopathic male infertility: what is the new evidence. Urology. 2015;86:1065-75.

Impact of Thyroid Autoimmunity on Outcomes of Assisted Reproduction

Ritu Hinduja

■ INTRODUCTION

The presence of antithyroid antibodies (ATAs) is recognized as thyroid autoimmunity (TAI), more specifically the presence of antithyroglobulin (anti-TG) and antithyroid peroxidase (anti-TPO) antibodies with a prevalence of 5–15%.[1] TAI is the most common autoimmune disorder in the women of reproductive age and its prevalence increases in the women suffering from infertility to a close of 10–31%.[2] TAI is known to be associated with numerous adverse obstetric outcomes like preterm delivery, placental abruption, and low birth weight.[3] There is a strong proven association of TAI with miscarriages, this relationship was first established in 1990 by Stagnaro-Green.[1] However, some studies subsequently refuted this association. Several studies did show a correlation between TAI and miscarriages in women who conceived spontaneously,[4,5] but this association in infertile women undergoing assisted reproductive technology (ART) treatments is still unclear.

Thyroid autoimmunity has been found to be related to subclinical hypothyroidism (SCH).[6-8]

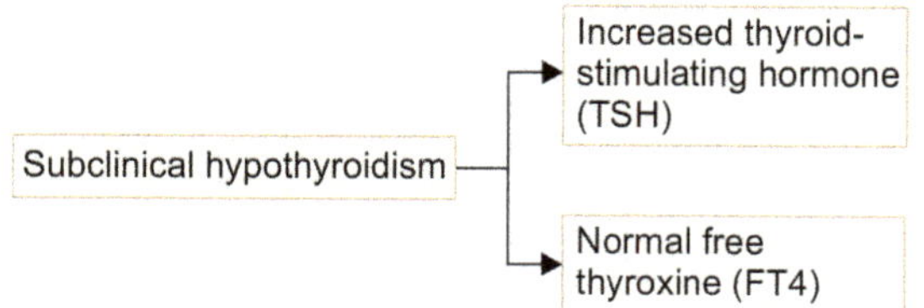

Several aspects of reproduction are affected by the disturbances in the thyroid function.[9,10] TAI in a euthyroid women is related to increased incidence of miscarriages and in the infertile women, TAI is seen to be more prevalent in women with endometriosis, tubal disease, and ovulatory dysfunction.[11-13] What still eludes us is the pathophysiology underlying the association between TAI and miscarriage.

Following three mechanisms can be hypothesized for the association:

1. An immune dysfunction.
2. A direct action of antithyroglobulin antibodies (TgAbs) on the placenta (this has been demonstrated in mice but not on humans).[14]
3. Decrease in the thyroid hormone in pregnant women with TAI.[15]

Thyroid gland, in particular, is under a lot of stress during pregnancy and trying to keep up with the increased demands of the thyroid hormone to suffice for birth, the mother, and the fetus. The few changes that affect the thyroid in pregnancy are as follows:

- Peaking of human chorionic gonadotropin (hCG) around the 8th–10th weeks of pregnancy.
- Increased levels of estrogen → Leads to an increase in serum thyroxine-binding globulin (TBG) concentrations → Causing reduction in FT4 and a compensatory increase in serum TSH.

However, unless the pregnancy is associated with iodine deficiency, both TSH and FT4 remain within their normal range.[16-18] Thyroid function is proven to be deranged by ovarian hyperstimulation.[19] Moreover, in the presence of positive anti-thyroid antibodies it was observed that serum TSH levels are increased in 16% of the women at delivery.[20] It has also been shown that TSH values prior to ART treatment, at 12 weeks and 30 weeks after conception, were all significantly higher in anti-TPO-positive women.[21]

It is hypothesized that if TAI affects pregnancy at every stage and even the levels before pregnancy play an important role, it must exert some effect on the ART cycles. This article explores those aspects.

The most popular hypothesis is that TAI exerts its effect in both a TSH-independent and TSH-dependent manner.[22]

Thyroid-stimulating hormone independent means that ATAs level may be an indication of autoimmune dysfunction such as increased endometrial T-cell population, hyperactivity, and elevated mass of natural killer cells and activated polyclonal B-cells. In ATA-positive women, the above mentioned immunological factors were activated, and attacked trophoblast-placental tissue, leading to miscarriage and fetal wastage. One study[23] concluded that ATAs interfere with fertilization and embryo development and implantation by binding to the surface of the egg and/or embryo or attacking the endometrium. However, there is limited evidence of a TSH-independent mechanism. As there is no dose-dependent effect demonstrated between the titers of the ATAs and miscarriage and the role of immunotherapy in prevention of miscarriages is also not proven. The effect of heparin/aspirin therapy alone versus heparin/aspirin in combination with intravenous immunoglobulin (IVIg) immunotherapy on *in vitro* fertilization (IVF) outcomes of patients with positive ATA was studied by Sher G et al.[24] The study found that IVIg was associated with increased live birth rate, but did not affect miscarriage rate.

It has been observed that TSH by increasing the proliferative capacity and activity of natural killer cells can stimulate the immune system, and this might be responsible for causing miscarriages.[25] Another assumption is that it is the high normal TSH values, rather than ATA levels that cause a miscarriage.

Because of the scarcity of information, the pathogenic mechanisms responsible for infertility in presence of ATA are largely speculative. The decrease in triiodothyronine (T3) concentrations, as sometimes occurs in women with positive TAI, may play a role in the following manner:

- On steroid biosynthesis, T3 modulates follicle-stimulating hormone (FSH) and luteinizing hormone (LH) action.
- In human oocyte, different isoforms of T3 receptors have been identified.

Thus, a decreased availability of T3 might impact the normal female reproductive function negatively. *The ovarian follicle* hypothesis was proposed by Monteleone et al. in which they demonstrated measurable amounts of ATAs in the follicular fluid obtained from women with ATA positive and these follicular levels strongly correlated with the blood serum levels. They also observed that women with ATA positive had a decreased fertilization rate and reduced number of good embryos available. Based on this, they hypothesized:

- Presence of thyroid antibody mediated cytotoxicity in the growing follicle may damage the maturing oocyte

Finally, thyroid-independent mechanisms involving abnormal innate and humoral immunity and vitamin D deficiency have been proposed to explain the association between TAI and fertility.

Vissenberg et al., in their interesting review, concluded that the presence of anti-TPO antibody (anti-TPOAb) negatively influences folliculogenesis, spermatogenesis, fertilization rates (FRs), embryo quality, and pregnancy rates. However, the pathophysiology behind it remains completely speculative, as the studies so far have been on animal models. In IVF, the effect of thyroid antibodies on each stage of reproductive process from the oocyte to the embryo can be studied and also the exact biochemical stage of pregnancy can also be precisely determined making it an excellent model to study the effect of TAI and its pathophysiology.

◼ EFFECT OF THYROID AUTOIMMUNITY ON OVARIAN RESERVE

Thyroid autoimmunity has been associated with decreased ovarian reserve by many authors. However, the underlying pathophysiology remains elusive. There have been theories proposed and one of them is that ovary shares multiple antigens with the thyroid gland and hence makes them venerable to the action of the ATAs.

In order to gain a deeper understanding, a large cross-sectional study was conducted by Polyzos et al. In this study, they evaluated the prevalence of positive anti-TPO antibodies in three groups of women defined according to the age-specific levels of anti-Müllerian hormone. They failed to demonstrate any association between TAI and decreased ovarian reserve. Since ovarian response to stimulation is considered a noninvasive surrogate measurement of ovarian reserve a comparable response to ovarian stimulation in terms of oocytes retrieved between patients with positive and negative TAI indirectly corroborates the results of Polyzos et al. These two conflicting results force us to speculate an all-or-none phenomenon. The negative effect of TAI on ovarian reserve may occur only in a small subset of women and may rapidly progress into a total exhaustion of the ovarian reserve. If this pathogenetic mechanism does not switch on, the ovarian reserve would remain intact. This would explain the higher frequency of TAI in women with premature ovarian failure (POF), but not in women with reduced ovarian reserve.

◼ EFFECT OF THYROID AUTOIMMUNITY ON FERTILIZATION

Monteleone et al. (2011) hypothesized that the lower fertilization rate, decreased embryo quality, and compromised implantation rate in women with positive ATAs may be because the thyroid antibodies may bind to the antigens expressed in the zona pellucida and destroy the important functional role of zona. Therefore, suggesting that intracytoplasmic sperm injection (ICSI) can overcome the negative effect of thyroid autoantibodies, unfortunately there is dearth of data supporting this.

EFFECT OF THYROID AUTOIMMUNITY ON IMPLANTATION

Weghofer et al. showed that, in women with low functional ovarian reserve, TPOAb significantly affected embryo quality in euthyroid women with low-normal TSH values (i.e. TSH ≤ 2.5 µIU/mL). In women with TPOAb and high-normal TSH levels, a trend toward impaired embryo quality, although not statistically significant (P = 0.056), was observed.

There is scanty evidence on the effect of TAI on the endometrium. Kilic et al. in his study evaluated the endometrial volume in TAI-positive and negative women with unexplained infertility and failed to demonstrate any correlation. The harmful effect of TPOAb and TgAb on the endometrial surface can be justified if the expression of TPO and Tg in the endometrium is demonstrated which is still a matter of debate. Furthermore, TPOAb might be able to recognize other proteins expressed in the uterus that belongs to the family of mammalian heme peroxidases such as prostaglandin G/H synthase 2 (PTGS2). Since PTGS2 is known to play a role in female fertility and given its importance for an ongoing pregnancy both in human and mice, one could speculate an effect of TPOAb on PTGS2 with a consequence on implantation. However, no data supporting this hypothesis are available.

OVARIAN HYPERSTIMULATION AND THYROID FUNCTION

Controlled ovarian hyperstimulation (COH) is the central process in IVF. Serum estradiol levels in these patients may increase and reach supraphysiologic levels approximately (4,000–6,000 ng/L). This high estrogen causes rise of thyroglobulin (TBG), which reduces free thyroid hormone causing positive feedback mechanism to further increase TSH levels. Human chorionic gonadotropin also has direct stimulatory effect on thyroid receptors, leading to increase in thyroid hormone and decreasing TSH.

The American Thyroid Association (ATA), 2017 guidelines recommend:
- As the interpretation of the TSH reports during COH is difficult, perform thyroid function testing before or 1–2 weeks after the stimulation.

- Thyroid function testing should be done in all pregnancies following COH.
  - Ideally, the reference range/values of thyroid function tests should be population and trimester-specific. This can be defined by the laboratory and should represent typical population of that region. This reference range should be defined in healthy TPOAb-negative pregnant women with optimal iodine intake and without thyroid illness.
  - If the reference range is not available, TSH assays performed in similar pregnant patient population can be used as reference.
  - If this is also not available, then generally an upper reference limit of TSH of 4.0 mU/L may be used. For most assays, this limit represents a reduction in the nonpregnant TSH upper reference limit of 0.5 mU/L.
- In women who are not pregnant, but have slightly raised TSH levels due to controlled ovarian stimulation, values should be repeated after 2–4 weeks. This is the time required for the hormones to reach baseline levels **(Table 1 and Flowchart 1)**.

TREATMENT STRATEGIES FOR THYROID AUTOIMMUNITY-POSITIVE WOMEN

Adequate treatment options for the harmful effect of TAI on pregnancy outcomes have not yet been established.

There are proposed strategies based on different presumed pathogenetic hypotheses:
- *Prescribing levothyroxine*: Assuming that the poor pregnancy and delivery outcome of TPOAb-positive women is due to a mild thyroid dysfunction.
- *Use of glucocorticoids*: It fits with the hypothesis that TAI could represent a marker of an underlying generalized autoimmune imbalance.

A study by Korevaar et al. on the relationship between the maternal thyroid function during early pregnancy and the intelligent quotient in the offspring and the brain morphology in childhood raises concerns regarding the overtreatment with T4 in the population. Therefore, the fraternity is use T4 with caution while using a strict cutoff threshold of 2.5 mIU/L of TSH as it may hold potential risks.

CONCLUSION

In conclusion, TAI does not hamper the outcomes of ART in women without SCH and the apparent correlation between TAI and miscarriage in women with unknown status of SCH may be because of some TSH-dependent pathophysiology or because of presence of SCH. Hence, it is recommended that women with TAI specially combined with SCH should be monitored carefully for the risk of

TABLE 1: Guidelines of international societies regarding investigation approaches in infertile women before or during pregnancy.

Society	Before ovarian stimulation	During ovarian stimulation	During (early) pregnancy
ASRM	It is rational to test TSH in infertile women planning conception	No recommendation	No recommendation
ATA	Women with infertility should have screening with TSH, as part of their infertility workup	There is insufficient evidence to recommend for or against screening for thyroid antibodies in women undergoing IVF	Serum TSH values should be obtained early in pregnancy in women at high risk for overt hypothyroidism (including those with infertility)
ES	Individuals at high risk for thyroid illness (including infertile women or those with a known thyroid disease) should be identified before pregnancy and TSH should be measured Universal screening for anti-TPO antibodies before pregnancy is not recommended	No recommendation	No agreement regarding screening recommendations for all newly pregnant women Universal screening for anti-TPO antibodies during pregnancy is not recommended
ETA	No recommendation	No recommendation	Evidence for screening for SCH in pregnancy is equivocal Trimester-specific reference ranges for TSH and T4 (total or free) should be established in each antenatal hospital setting. If not available, the following reference range of upper limits are recommended: first trimester 2.5 mIU/mL, second trimester 3.0 mIU/mL, and third trimester 3.5 mIU/mL In hypothyroid women already treated with LT4 before conception, TSH should be checked every 4–6 weeks during the first trimester and once during the second and third trimesters

(anti-TPO: antithyroid peroxidase; ASRM: American Society for Reproductive Medicine; ATA: American Thyroid Association; ES: Endocrine Society; ETA: European Thyroid Association; IVF: *in vitro* fertilization; LT4: levothyroxine; SCH: subclinical hypothyroidism; T4: thyroxine; TSH: thyroid-stimulating hormone)

TABLE 2: Summary of the available evidence on thyroid hormones and the effect on reproduction[26]

Thyroid hormones	
Oocytes and ovulation	Thyroid hormone disorders are associated with disturbed folliculogenesis T3 in combination with FSH enhances granulosa cell proliferation and inhibits granulosa cell apoptosis by the PI3K/Akt pathway Thyroid hormone transporters and receptors are expressed in the ovary
Sperm	Hypothyroidism has an adverse effect on human spermatogenesis and negatively affects sperm count and motility as well as morphology Hyperthyroidism is associated with abnormalities in sperm motility and DNA damage No studies are available on the mechanisms by which thyroid hormone affects spermatogenesis
Fertilization and embryogenesis	Hypothyroidism is associated with lower fertilization rates and disturbed embryogenesis No studies on the pathophysiology have been reported
Endometrium	Deiodinases, THRA and THRB are expressed in the endometrium Evidence for a direct effect of thyroid hormone on endometrial receptivity or function is lacking
Implantation	Thyroid hormone stimulates the production of progesterone in granulosa cells and up-regulates L1F There are no studies on the effect of thyroid hormone on implantation
Placentation	T3 increases the expression of MMP-2, MMP-3, fetal fibronectin and integrin $\alpha5\beta1$T3 in early placental extravillous trophoblasts

T3, triiodothyronine; THRA, thyroid hormone receptor alpha; THRB, thyroid hormone receptor beta; L1F, leukemia inhibiting factor; MMP-2,3, matrix metalloproteinase 2,3.

Flowchart 1: Effect of thyroid autoimmunity on different parameters summarized.

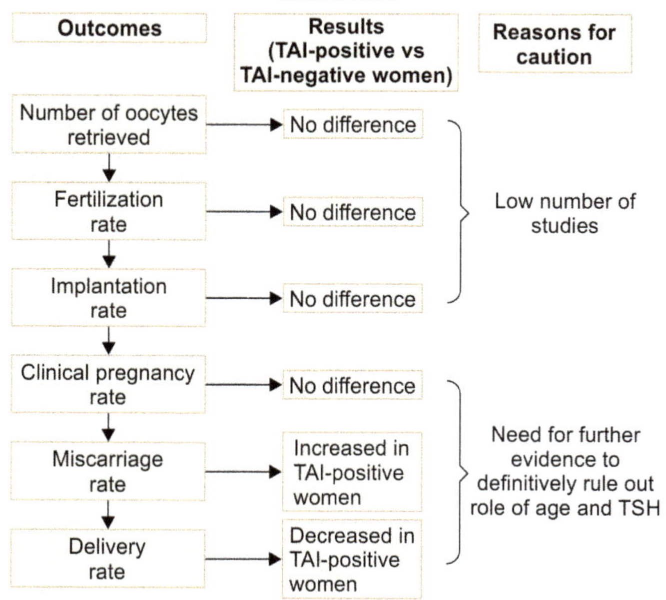

(TAI: thyroid autoimmunity; TSH: thyroid-stimulating hormone)

TABLE 3: Summary of the available evidence on thyroid peroxidase autoantibodies (TPO-Ab) and the effect on reproduction.[26]

TPO-Antibodies

Oocytes and ovulation	TPO-Ab are present in follicular fluid TPO-Ab do not influence the number of retrieved oocytes during controlled ovarian stimulation There are no studies on a direct effect of TPO-Ab on folliculogenesis
Sperm	TPO-Ab are more often found in subfertile men compared with a control group. No studies are available that showing a direct effect of TPO-Ab on spermatogenesis
Fertilization and embryogenesis	TPO-Ab are associated with lower fertilization rates and disturbed embryogenesis No literature is available on the pathophysiology
Endometrium	TPO-Ab do not influence endometrial volume No studies have been published on direct effects of TPO-Ab on endometrial receptivity or endometrial function
Implantation	There are no studies on direct effects of TPO-Ab on implantation
Placentation	TPO-Ab diffuse through the placental barrier There is no evidence for a direct effect of TPO-Ab on early placentation

miscarriage. These conclusions are of great value, however, there are still studies that are required to explore not only the fundamentals but also to gain deep insight in the pathophysiology backing this entire phenomenon. The interesting association between TAI and decreased ovarian reserve is worth researching more about. Another interesting study would be comparing the outcomes of IVF versus ICSI in women with TAI-positive status. Finally, evidence of the effect of TAI on endometrial receptivity and embryo implantation is particularly lacking. Given the complexity of the process, every factor involved, starting with the quality of the embryo to the endometrial receptivity, should be studied separately.

The impact of TAI on outcomes of assisted reproduction is an iceberg and we have not even scratched the surface of its tip.

REFERENCES

1. Stagnaro-Green A, Roman SH, Cobin RH, et al. Detection of at-risk pregnancy by means of highly sensitive assays for thyroid autoantibodies. JAMA. 1990;264:1422-5.
2. Glinoer D, de Nayer P, Bourdoux P, et al. Regulation of maternal thyroid during pregnancy. J Clin Endocrinol Metab. 1990;71:276-87.
3. Chan S, Boelaert K. Optimal management of hypothyroidism, hypothyroxinaemia and euthyroid TPO antibody positivity preconception and in pregnancy. Clin Endocrinol. 2015;82:313-26.
4. Chen L, Hu R. Thyroid autoimmunity and miscarriage: a meta-analysis. Clin Endocrinol. 2011;74:513-9.
5. van den Boogaard E, Vissenberg R, Land JA, et al. Significance of (sub)clinical thyroid dysfunction and thyroid autoimmunity before conception and in early pregnancy: a systematic review. Hum Reprod Update. 2011;17:605-19.
6. Johnson N, Chatrani V, Taylor-Christmas AK, et al. Population reference values and prevalence rates following universal screening for subclinical hypothyroidism during pregnancy of an Afro-Caribbean cohort. Eur Thyroid J. 2014;3:234-9.
7. McElduff A, Morris J. Thyroid function tests and thyroid autoantibodies in an unselected population of women undergoing first trimester screening for aneuploidy. Aust N Z J Obstet Gynaecol. 2008;48:478-80.
8. Chai J, Yeung WY, Lee CY, et al. Live birth rates following in vitro fertilization in women with thyroid autoimmunity and/or subclinical hypothyroidism. Clin Endocrinol. 2013;80:122-7.
9. Krassas GE. Thyroid disease and female reproduction. Fertil Steril. 2000;74:1063-70.
10. Poppe K, Glinoer D. Thyroid autoimmunity and hypothyroidism before and during pregnancy. Hum Reprod Update. 2003;9:149-61.
11. Abramson J, Stagnaro-Green A. Thyroid antibodies and fetal loss: an evolving story. Thyroid. 2001;11:57-63.
12. Poppe K, Glinoer D, Tournaye H, et al. Assisted reproduction and thyroid autoimmunity: an unfortunate combination? J Clin Endocrinol Metab. 2003;88:4149-52.
13. Poppe K, Glinoer D, Van Steirteghem A, et al. Thyroid dysfunction and autoimmunity in infertile women. Thyroid. 2002;12:997-1001.
14. Matalon ST, Blank M, Levy Y, et al. The pathogenic role of anti-thyroglobulin antibody on pregnancy: evidence from an active immunization model in mice. Hum Reprod. 2003;18:1094-9.
15. Maruo T, Katayama K, Matuso H, et al. The role of maternal thyroid hormones in maintaining early pregnancy in threatened abortion. Acta Endocrinol (Copenh). 1992;127:118-22.
16. Glinoer D. The regulation of thyroid function in pregnancy: pathways of endocrine adaptation from physiology to pathology. Endocr Rev. 1997;18:404-33.
17. Glinoer D, Delange F. The potential repercussions of maternal, fetal, and neonatal hypothyroxinemia on the progeny. Thyroid. 2000;10:871-87.

18. Glinoer D, De Nayer P, Delange F, et al. A randomized trial for the treatment of mild iodine deficiency during pregnancy: maternal and neonatal effects. J Clin Endocrinol Metab. 1995;80:258-69.

19. Muller AF, Verhoeff A, Mantel MJ, et al. Decrease of free thyroxine levels after controlled ovarian hyperstimulation. J Clin Endocrinol Metab. 2000;85:545-8.

20. Glinoer D, Riahi M, Grun JP, et al. Risk of subclinical hypothyroidism in pregnant women with asymptomatic autoimmune thyroid disorders. J Clin Endocrinol Metab. 1994;79:197-204.

21. Negro R, Formoso G, Coppola L, et al. Euthyroid women with autoimmune disease undergoing assisted reproduction technologies: the role of autoimmunity and thyroid function. J Endocrinol Invest. 2007;30:3-8.

22. Twig G, Shina A, Amital H, et al. Pathogenesis of infertility and recurrent pregnancy loss in thyroid autoimmunity. J Autoimmun. 2012;38:J275-81.

23. Zhong YP, Ying Y, Wu HT, et al. Relationship between antithyroid antibody and pregnancy outcome following in vitro fertilization and embryo transfer. Int J Med Sci. 2012;9:121-5.

24. Sher G, Maassarani G, Zouves C, et al. The use of combined heparin/aspirin and immunoglobulin G therapy in the treatment of in vitro fertilization patients with antithyroid antibodies. Am J Reprod Immunol. 1998;39:223-5.

25. Provinciali M, Di Stefano G, Fabris N. Improvement in the proliferative capacity and natural killer cell activity of murine spleen lymphocytes by thyrotropin. Int J Immunopharmacol. 1992;14:865-70.

26. https://academic.oup.com/humupd/article/21/3/378/676494

Surgery as Adjuvant in Infertility

S Krishnakumar, Rohan Krishnakumar

■ INTRODUCTION

Infertility is a rising pandemic. It has far reaching consequences on the mental, social, and psychological well-being of a couple. Advances in assisted reproductive technology (ART) have improved the fertility outcome in despondent cases. Fertility enhancing surgeries are a major component of infertility treatment and aim to optimize the results of the treatment. Fertility enhancing surgeries may be used to aid natural conception or as an adjuvant method prior to performing *in vitro* fertilization (IVF). While data suggesting surgery for hydrosalpinx prior to ART treatment is robust, surgery for other indications like fibroids, polyps, uterine anomalies, and Asherman is controversial and lacks strong evidence.

This chapter aims to highlight some of the surgical procedures commonly performed to improve the fertility outcomes both naturally and in ART.

■ FERTILITY ENHANCING SURGERIES THAT AID IN NATURAL CONCEPTION

Certain uterine or tubal factors like myoma, polyps, tubal obstruction or adhesions can cause a hindrance in natural conception. Surgery can correct this pathology and help achieve a natural pregnancy.

The following procedures are mainstay to help achieve a natural conception:

- *Uterine myomas*: Laparoscopic or hysteroscopic myomectomy
- Uterine polyp
- *Proximal tubal occlusion*: Tubal cannulation
- *Distal tubal obstruction*: Adhesiolysis and tubal reconstruction

- *Laparoscopic ovarian drilling*: Anovulation
- *Endometriosis*: Adhesiolysis, endometrioma cystectomy or ablation and drainage.

■ TUBAL FACTOR

Tubal factor accounts for 25–35% of infertility cases. Proximal tubal obstruction is more common than distal. Proximal blockage may be due to obstruction caused by mucus plugs or debris, tubal spasm or occlusion (anatomical blockage). Tubal occlusion commonly occurs as a result of fibrosis either due to infection or endometriosis. Tubal obstruction is generally treatable with a simple cannulation and has shown promising results. Cannulation is performed via a coaxial catheter usually guided hysteroscopically with simultaneous visualization via laparoscopy. Contraindications to the procedure include active genital infection, suspected pregnancy or malignancy.[1] Tubal cannulation has shown successful results in 85% cases with bilateral tubal block and 95% in unilateral block, while pregnancy was achieved in 30–50% of the cases only. In patients who do not conceive within 6 months of tubal cannulation, the option of IVF must be considered soon.

However, in cases of tubal occlusion or in some cases of distal tubal block, tubal microsurgical procedures may be useful. For proximal tubal occlusion, tubocornual anastomosis can be used to restore tubal patency. Indications for tubal microsurgery include:

- Tubal sterilization reversal
- Mid-tubal block
- Salpingitis isthmica nodosa.

The principle of tubal microsurgery is to treat pelvic adhesions and restore the normal tubo-ovarian anatomy.

Microsurgery needs a certain degree of expertise. The aim of the surgery is to minimize tissue damage and ensure proper healing of the tissue to prevent adhesions.

Distal obstruction is commonly caused by either hydrosalpinx or fimbrial phimosis. Management of hydrosalpinx will be discussed elsewhere in the chapter. In cases of fimbrial phimosis, a fimbrioplasty may be attempted.

MYOMAS

Myoma is benign hypertrophy of uterine musculature. They are a common cause for infertility. The International Federation of Gynecology and Obstetrics (FIGO) classification divides fibroids/myomas into eight subgroups. Submucosal and intramural fibroids are implicated as a cause of infertility and have in some circumstances caused pregnancy loss. The routine approach of myomectomy for patients undergoing infertility treatment is controversial. The number, site, and size of the fibroid are critical in deciding the line of management.

Which Fibroids Need to be Operated?[2]

- Any fibroid which is symptomatic (menstrual abnormalities and pressure symptoms)
- Presence of submucosal or intramural fibroids that distort uterine cavity
- Intramural fibroids >5 cm
- Multiple fibroids
- Recurrent implantation failure.

HYSTEROSCOPIC MYOMECTOMY

Submucous myomas are divided into FIGO group 0, 1, and 2. These fibroids may alter the endometrial receptivity and also impair endometrial contractility, thus contributing to infertility. Group 0 and 1 myomas are generally treated via hysteroscopic myomectomy. A thorough preoperative evaluation is done. Correction of anemia is important. In cases with large fibroids, preoperative gonadotropin-releasing hormone (GnRH) agonist may help to decrease the size and vascularity. Vercellini in a study reported 49%, 36%, and 33% fertility rates over 3-year period for type 0, 1, and 2 of fibroids.[3] Techniques for hysteroscopic myomectomy include following.

Resectoscope

Traditionally, resectoscope was the standard instrument use for resecting a submucous myoma. Bipolar electrode is preferred over unipolar electrode owing to its greater safety margin.

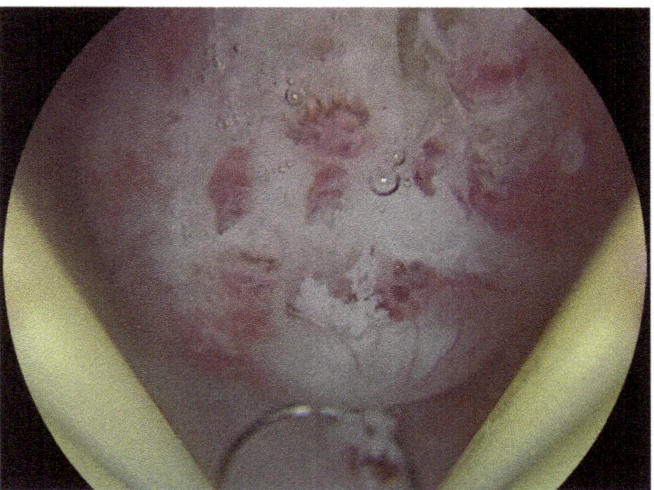

Fig. 1: Hysteroscopic resection of submucous myoma.

Hysteroscopic Morcellator (Fig. 1)

Advancement in technology has enabled the use of mechanical energy for fibroid resection. Morcellator provide the advantage of avoiding complications of fluid overload and electrosurgical complications; however, the modality is expensive.

Complications of hysteroscopic myomectomy are as follows:
- Postoperative bleeding
- Fluid intravasation syndrome
- Electrosurgical complications
- Asherman's syndrome.

LAPAROSCOPIC MYOMECTOMY

This is the preferred route for surgery in case of multiple fibroids or large intramural fibroids. Proper preoperative mapping is crucial to decide the number and site of incisions. Use of vasopressin helps decrease the blood loss during surgery. Enucleation and suturing the myoma bed are the most important steps of surgery. Delayed absorbable sutures are generally preferred. Excessive use of electrocautery must be avoided to avoid necrosis of tissue.

Role of myomectomy prior to IVF is debatable. A comparative analysis reported about the effectiveness of myomectomy prior to IVF. Patients selected were diagnosed with intramural-subserosal fibroids, with at least one lesion with a mean diameter of 5 cm. The groups were selected by the patients themselves. The cumulative delivery rate in women who did and did not undergo surgery was 25% and 12%, respectively.[4]

Role of myomectomy in unexplained infertility is controversial. However, several uncontrolled studies have shown pregnancy rates ranging between 44% and 62% after myomectomy.

■ UTERINE FACTORS: MÜLLERIAN ANOMALIES

Müllerian anomalies are anatomical defects that occur due to fusion defects of the müllerian ducts and can result in infertility. These contribute to almost 5–12% cases of infertility, of which uterine septum is the most commonly encountered anomaly accounting to 80–90%. Hysteroscopy forms the mainstay of treating intrauterine pathology. It is referred to as the "see and treat" technique since it provides the advantage of simultaneously diagnosis and treatment.[5]

Uterine Septum (Figs. 2A and B)

The septate uterus is the most common form of congenital malformation that may result in repeated pregnancy loss and infertility. According to European Society of Human Reproduction and Embryology (ESHRE) classification, septate uterus (class U2) is defined as the one with an internal indentation >50% of uterine wall thickness with an external contour that is straight or has indentation of <50%. They are further subclassified into partial and complete septum.

There may occur concomitant cervical or vaginal septum. Most of these patients are asymptomatic and anomalies are detected on workup for recurrent pregnancy loss.

When to Perform a Hysteroscopic Septoplasty?

There is insufficient evidence to support the need of septal resection in all patients, especially if incidentally diagnosed on imaging. However, in patients with history of repeated abortions, septal resection has shown to improve the chances of pregnancy.

Management

There is no conclusive evidence supporting septal resection in every case of infertility; however, multiple studies have claimed that septal resection improves chances of pregnancy. Also, in patients with history of recurrent pregnancy loss, septoplasty has proven to be beneficial.

Methods for septal resection include cold scissors, needle electrodes or transcervical resection using Collins knife resectoscope. The scissors are mostly preferred in cases of partial septum. In broad, thick, and complete septum, a resectoscope is a better method. The septum is a fibroelastic tissue which is avascular and retracts upon dissection.

There is no evidence to suggest the best time to conceive after a septal resection; however, a study conducted for a second look postseptoplasty showed complete healing of the cavity in 8 weeks.[6]

Hysteroscopic Lateral Metroplasty

This is a fertility improving surgery done in cases with abnormal shape of the uterine cavity, especially in the T-shaped uterus. Dysmorphic (T-shaped uterus), traditionally categorized as class VII, are now considered in class U1 of the ESHRE classification. The exact mechanism contributing to infertility is yet unknown. However, it is postulated that an altered volume and shape of the uterine cavity may affect the endometrial receptivity thus affecting the fertility. Although considered a congenital anomaly, few cases may be acquired due to tuberculosis or Asherman's syndrome.

Indications

- T-shaped uterine cavity with a history of infertility or adverse pregnancy outcome
- In patients who have a failed In Vitro Fertilization and Embryo Transfer (IVF-ET) treatment.

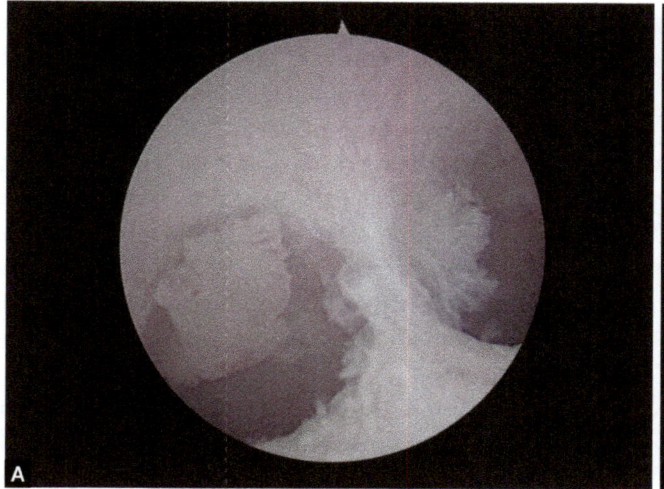
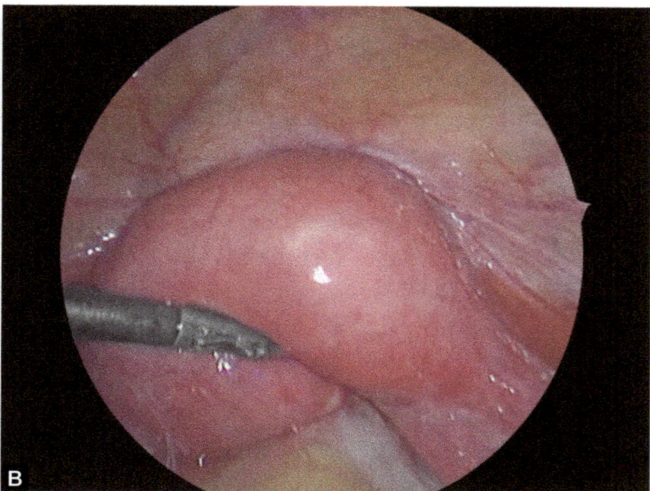

Figs. 2A and B: Uterine septum and laparoscopic confirmation of broad fundus.

Management

The surgery is generally performed in the immediate postmenstrual period to avoid a thickened endometrium of the luteal phase. The prerequisties of surgery are same as any other hysteroscopic procedure. The methods utilized for metroplasty include the scissors or a resectoscope with monopolar hook or bipolar electrode. The aim of surgery is to restore a triangular shape to the uterine cavity. The end point of metroplasty is considered when both the ostia are visualized from the level of the internal os.

ASHERMAN'S SYNDROME

Asherman's syndrome is a condition characterized by formation of intrauterine adhesions, occurring due to damage to the basal layer of endometrium. It is seen commonly postcurettage. Patients commonly present with symptoms of hypomenorrhea or amenorrhea and infertility. Although surgery improves the normal anatomy of the cavity, it has not proven to improve the endometrial vascularity. Depending on the severity they are classified as mild, moderate or severe degree of Asherman. It is preferable to perform adhesiolysis prior to initiating infertility treatment. Most patients require IVF since chances of natural conception in this subgroup of patients is dismal.

Adhesiolysis is commonly done using cold scissors in the mild or moderate group **(Fig. 3)**. However, in patients with severe degree of adhesions use of electrosurgery may be mandated. It is important to avoid overzealous adhesiolysis especially anatomical landmarks are distorted since it may lead to uterine perforation. A relook hysteroscopy is advised in such cases after 6 weeks to assess the cavity and complete the procedure. The rate of readhesion formation remains high ranging between 3.1% and 23.5%.[7] Certain measures can be taken for prevention of readhesion formation like use of mechanical balloon or use of hormonal medications.

The delivery rate post-treatment varied greatly in various studies and was directly proportional to the severity of the disease process. A study by Roy KK and Yu D et al. showed a delivery rate varying between 59% and 61% within 1 year and 87.2% and 97% within 2 years after spacing between hysteroscopic and adhesiolysis.[8] Adhesions caused as a result of genital tuberculosis are more difficult to treat. Owing to damage caused to the basal endometrium, pregnancy rates are poor.

POSTOPERATIVE MANAGEMENT IN HYSTEROSCOPIC SURGERIES

Prophylactic antibiotics are given to prevent infection. Use of mechanical barrier's like intrauterine balloon for prevention of intrauterine adhesions is controversial. In patients with concurrent septal resection, or profound adhesiolysis, a pediatric Foley catheter can be inserted for a period of 5–7 days. Most surgeons prefer use of cyclical estrogen and progesterone for promoting endometrial growth. Routine use of hormones for improving vascularization and re-epithelization of endometrial part is controversial. However, most clinicians prefer to give a combined estrogen and progesterone regimen for 2–3 months.

UTERINE POLYPS (FIG. 4)

Endometrial polyps are benign outgrowth of endometrial mucosa. Most polyps are asymptomatic; however, may present with heavy menstrual bleeding and pain. Polyps greater than 1.5 cm and in the upper part of uterine cavity can interfere with fertility. Polyps are postulated to interfere mechanically, they may alter the expression of molecular

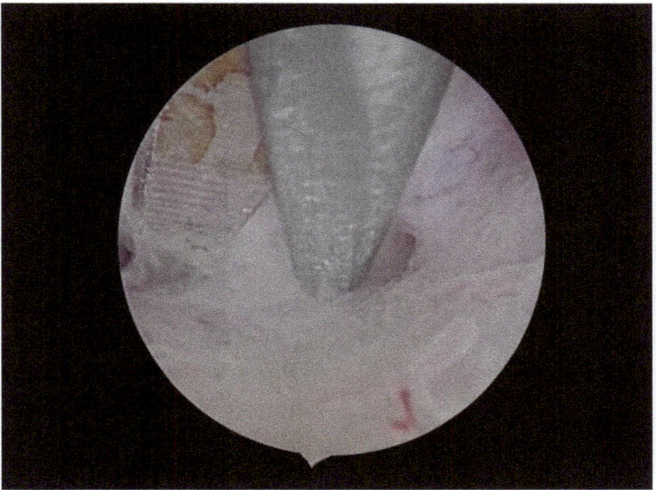

Fig. 3: Adhesiolysis with scissors in a case of Asherman's syndrome.

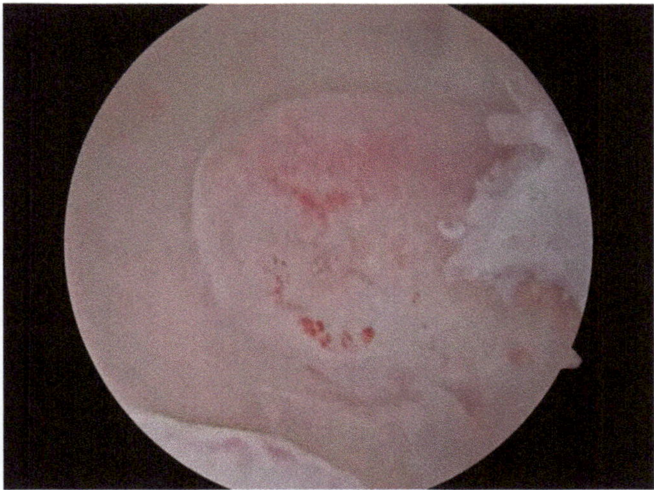

Fig. 4: Presence of uterine polyp arising from left lateral wall.

markers, *HOXA10* and *HOXA11* gene, and thus impair endometrial receptivity.[9,10]

All symptomatic polyps need to be excised. For asymptomatic polyps, several randomized controlled studies have shown benefit of polypectomy in otherwise unexplained infertility. Polypectomy may be performed with cold scissors, grasper or in case of large polyps resectoscope or morcellator may be required.

Treatment of polyps found incidentally during IVF stimulation is controversial. They may be excised whilst the cycle, or excised and planned for frozen embryo transfer or cycle cancelled. A study conducted by Lass et al. on a group of 83 women undergoing IVF with polyps detected incidentally (<2 cm) on ultrasonography (USG), were divided into two groups. Forty-nine women completed the standard IVF and embryo transfer treatment, and 34 women underwent hysteroscopic polypectomy immediately after oocyte retrieval and the embryos were cryopreserved and transferred in a subsequent cycle. There was no statistically significant difference in pregnancy rates in the two groups compared to overall fertility of patients visiting the clinic. However, a higher trend of pregnancy loss was noted in the fresh embryo transfer group.[11]

◼ LAPAROSCOPIC DRILLING OF POLYCYSTIC OVARIES (FIG. 5)

Laparoscopic ovarian drilling is a second-line method for management for infertile polycystic ovary disease (PCOD) patients. It is a safe and effective alternative to gonadotropin therapy. It achieves the same clinical pregnancy rate and live birth rate as gonadotropins and ensures mono-ovulation surpassing the side effect of ovarian hyperstimulation seen commonly with gonadotropins.

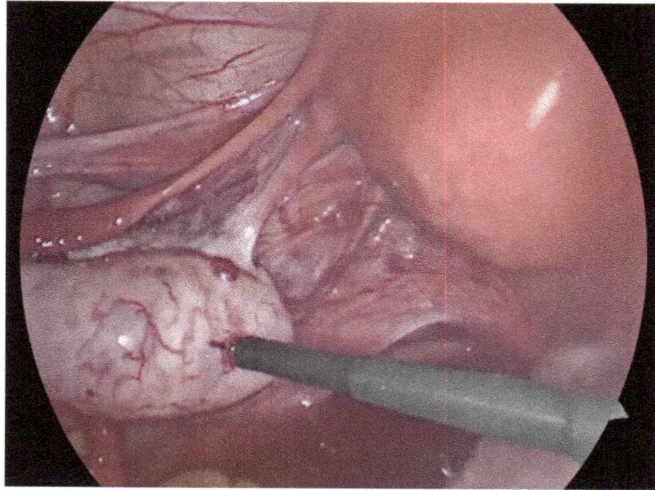

Fig. 5: Laparoscopic drilling of polycystic ovaries.

Indications

- Polycystic ovarian syndrome (PCOS) patients resistant to clomiphene citrate (CC)
- Patients with hypersecretion of luteinizing hormone (LH) with normal body mass index
- Patients requiring laparoscopy for other indications
- Alternative to gonadotropins where multiple pregnancy or ovarian hyperstimulation syndrome (OHSS) is a risk to the patient.

Procedure

This procedure is performed in selected group of patients as mentioned above. Generally, 3–8 punctures are performed via electrosurgery in each ovary using 600–800 J energy. This can result in normal ovulation in 74% of cases within 6 months.[12] More than 8 punctures are known to increase the incidence of postoperative pelvic adhesions and decrease the ovarian reserve.

A study conducted by Fernandez et al. concluded that ovarian drilling leads to spontaneous restoration of fertility in 20–64% of women with PCOS who had previously been infertile as a result of anovulation and who did not respond to CC treatment.[13]

◼ ENDOMETRIOSIS

Endometriosis affects 20–40% of women with history of subfertility. The possible reasons for subfertility in endometriosis include dyspareunia, alterations in pelvic anatomy, peritoneal or tubal adhesions, immunological factors, interference with fertilization, oocyte and embryo development, and implantation. The clinical presentation of the disease varies and the severity of symptoms may not necessarily correlate with the disease process. The disease process may be broadly categorized as:

- Superficial endometriosis
- Deep endometriosis
- Endometrioma.

The management approach for patients with infertility depends on the age of patient, duration of infertility, previous reproductive history, and presence of other infertility factors. The two broad spectrum fertility options include surgery followed by natural conception or IVF. In patients with no other obvious cause for infertility, surgery may be the mainstay. The Endometriosis Canadian (ENDOCAN) a multicenter randomized controlled trial (RCT) showed a twofold increase in conception rate following laparoscopy and treatment of superficial endometriosis compared with diagnostic laparoscopy alone. Endometriomas <4 cm may be managed conservatively.[14] However, in symptomatic patients surgery in the form of cystectomy or drainage and ablation maybe required. Long-term use of medical therapy postsurgery for suppression of disease process remains debatable. In infertile women with laparoscopy staged and confirmed endometriosis with no other infertility factors, the spontaneous pregnancy rate after expectant management is just 30% (moderate endometriosis) or 0% (severe endometriosis).[15]

The role of management of endometrioma prior to ART [particularlyintrauterine insemination (IUI)] remains controversial. It is proposed that the risk of physical reduction in ovarian reserve is greater with excision than with simple drainage and ablative therapy of endometrioma. A pooled analysis of RCTs favors excision in order to improve the chance of natural conception, to decrease recurrence of disease process, and reduce recurrence rate of symptoms. Currently available evidence is unclear whether endometrioma-related ovarian damage precedes or follows surgery. Most clinicians would recommend surgery followed by natural conception or to proceed with IVF in women with endometriomas.

Surgical Approach to Endometriosis (Figs. 6A and B)

- *In minimal-mild endometriosis*: Ablation of endometriotic lesions plus adhesiolysis to improve fertility is effective compared to diagnostic laparoscopy alone.
- *In moderate-severe endometriosis*: There is no consensus to one particular form of treatment. Adhesiolysis to restore normal pelvic anatomy is suggested.
- Laparoscopic cystectomy for ovarian endometriomas >4 cm diameter improves fertility compared to drainage and coagulation.
- Coagulation or laser vaporization of endometriomas without excision of the pseudocapsule is associated with a significantly increased risk of cyst recurrence.

In women with moderate-to-severe endometriosis, there are no controlled studies comparing reproductive outcome after surgery and after expectant management. The recommendations are based on evidence from two high-quality prospective cohort studies showing crude spontaneous pregnancy rates of 57–69% (moderate endometriosis) and 52–68% (severe endometriosis) after laparoscopic surgery, and on evidence from one high-quality prospective cohort study showing much lower crude pregnancy rates after expectant management: 33% (moderate endometriosis) and 0% (severe endometriosis).[16,17] A study by Nezhat and Vercellini has shown cumulative spontaneous pregnancy rate within 3 years after surgery to range between 46% and 77% for moderate endometriosis and between 44% and 74% for severe endometriosis.[16,17]

Overall, these data suggest that laparoscopic surgery is effective for the treatment of infertility associated with moderate-to-severe endometriosis. In patients with ovarian endometrioma, excision of endometrioma capsule increases the postoperative spontaneous pregnancy rate, compared to drainage and electrocoagulation of the endometrioma wall.[18] However, both techniques carry potential risks for reducing the ovarian reserve.

In vitro fertilization should be considered in patients with tubal damage, associated male factor infertility and if previous fertility treatment has failed. In patients with moderate-severe endometriosis, treatment with GnRH agonists 2–3 months prior to IVF has shown to improve pregnancy rates.[19] Literature on treatment of endometrioma prior to IVF is sparse. The only published RCT on management of endometrioma prior to IVF failed to show significant differences in fertilization, implantation, and pregnancy rates in 99 women allocated to either surgery or no surgery. Surgery; however, resulted in significantly

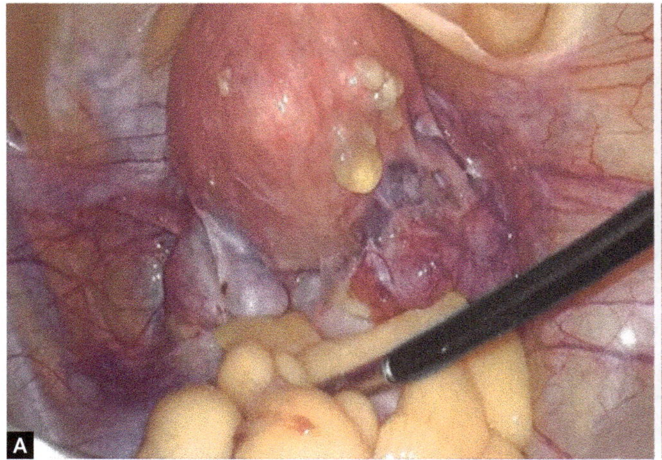
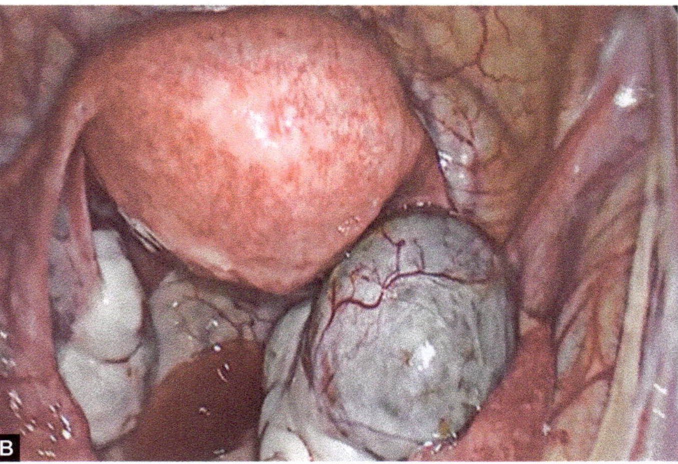

Figs. 6A and B: Depicting grade 4 endometriosis and large endometriotic cyst on right side.

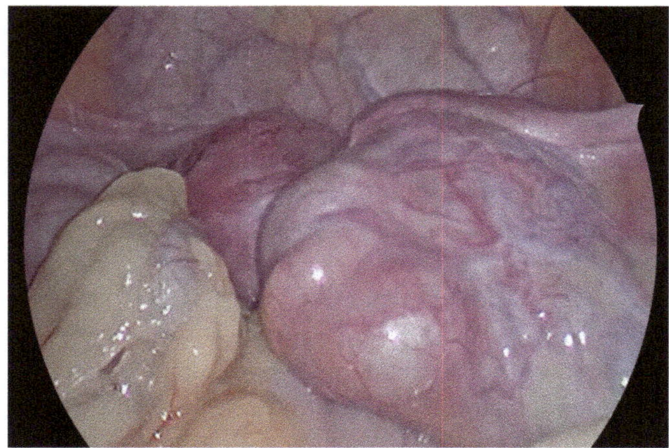

Fig. 7: Bilateral hydrosalpinx.

longer stimulation, higher follicle-stimulating hormone requirements, and lower oocyte numbers.[20]

FERTILITY-ENHANCING SURGERIES—ADJUVANT PRIOR TO IVF

Routine application of fertility enhancing surgeries is not recommended in all patients undergoing IVF treatment. However, in certain situations, surgery might aid to improve the results of infertility treatment especially when undergoing IVF. Some of these conditions have been highlighted below.

Hydrosalpinx (Fig. 7)

Hydrosalpinx is a pathological condition involving fluid accumulation in the fallopian tubes often as a result of chronic inflammation caused by prior sexually transmitted infections. Several retrospective analytical studies have proven the deleterious effect of hydrosalpinx on ART.[21,22] It is claimed that the chances of achieving pregnancy are halved and the incidence of spontaneous abortion are almost doubled in cases of proven hydrosalpinx.

The fluid accumulated in the tubes is considered to be embryotoxic, which may have a deleterious effect on the pregnancy. Hence, many treatment options like tubal ligation or clipping, aspiration of hydrosalpinx fluid or salpingectomy are being considered before proceeding with ART. The literature regarding the best method to achieve the same is sparse and inconclusive. While salpingectomy seems to be the best solution to hydrosalpinx, this surgery is not a standard procedure for all cases owing to concerns of damaging the ovarian blood supply. However, in grade 3 hydrosalpinx, salpingectomy does have a role in treatment.[23]

Tubal delinking is a popular alternative to salpingectomy. The procedure involves cauterizing the cornual ends of both the fallopian tubes, which is believed to prevent the backward flow of the toxic fluid. Hence, this has a positive effect on pregnancy rate post-ART. The role of ultrasound-guided drainage of hydrosalpinx during oocyte retrieval is unproven. In 2010 Cochrane analysis of five RCT over surgical management of tubal disease prior to IVF, results following laparoscopic salpingectomy, tubal occlusion, and USG aspiration were studied. They found that ongoing pregnancy rates and clinical pregnancy rates were improved in the salpingectomy group prior to IVF.[24]

Endometrial Scratching

Endometrial scratching is an experimental procedure. It involves taking a small biopsy of the endometrium, or making few cuts over the endometrium. It is said to be beneficial in the subgroup of patients who have repeated implantation failure. It is postulated that endometrial injury caused by this method, induces inflammatory, and immunological mechanisms that may aid in implantation. Endometrial scratching upregulates certain endometrial genes like mucin 1, transmembrane, alpha-crystallin B, phospholipase A2, etc.[25]

Although there is no conclusive evidence to suggest scratching in every couple undergoing IVF, multiple randomized studies have shown a positive outcome in patients with recurrent implantation failure. It is preferable to avoid doing the procedure simultaneously with oocyte retrieval since it is associated with reduced clinical and ongoing pregnancy rates.[26]

A Cochrane review indicated that endometrial scratching performed between Day 7 of previous cycle and Day 7 of embryo transfer cycle improves live birth and clinical pregnancy rates in patients with previous two failed embryo transfer. However, all evidence is moderate quality and involves a diverse heterogeneous group of patients and hence routine use of this procedure is not warranted in every case of implantation failure.[27]

CONCLUSION

In today's era of late marriages, couples are more career driven and opt for fertility at advanced age. Hence there is an alarming rise in the number of couples seeking fertility treatment. A thorough evaluation and workup is important to individualize the treatment plan for each patient. The spectrum of surgeries for the treatment of infertility varies widely. There is no standard protocol for all patients. The choice of surgery has to be individualized depending upon the characteristics of the disease process.

REFERENCES

1. Honoré GM, Holden AE, Schenken RS. Pathophysiology and management of proximal tubal blockage, Fertil Steril. 1999;71(5):785-95.

2. Ezzati M, Norian JM, Segars JH. Management of uterine fibroids in the patient pursuing assisted reproductive technologies. Womens Health (Lond). 2009;5:413-21.

3. Vercellini P, Zàina B, Yaylayan L, et al. Hysteroscopic myomectomy: Long term effects on menstrual pattern and fertility. Obstet Gynecol. 1999;94:341-7.

4. Bulletti C, De Ziegler D, Levi Setti P, et al. Myomas, pregnancy outcome, and in vitro fertilization. Ann N Y Acad Sci. 2004;1034:84-92.

5. Bettocchi S, Achilarre MT, Ceci O, et al. Fertility-enhancing hysteroscopic surgery. Semin Reprod Med. 2011;29(2):75-82.

6. Yang JH, Chen MJ, Chen CD, et al. Optimal waiting period for subsequent fertility treatment after various hysteroscopic surgeries. Fertil Steril. 2013;99(7):2092-6.

7. Yu D, Li TC, Xia E, et al. Factors affecting reproductive outcome of hysteroscopic adhesiolysis for Asherman's syndrome. Fertil Steril. 2008;89(3):715-22.

8. Roy KK, Baruah J, Sharma JB, et al. Reproductive outcome following hysteroscopic adhesiolysis in patients with infertility due to Asherman's syndrome. Arch Gynecol Obstet. 2010;281(2):355-61.

9. Spiewankiewicz B, Stelmachow J, Sawicki W, et al. The effectiveness of hysteroscopic polypectomy in cases of female infertility. Clin Exp Obstet Gynecol. 2003;30:23-5.

10. Shokeir TA, Shalan HM, El-Shafei MM. Significance of endometrial polyps detected hysteroscopically in eumenorrheic infertile women. J Obstet Gynecol Res. 2004;30:84-9.

11. Lass A, Williams G, Abusheikha N, et al. The effect of endometrial polyps on outcomes of in vitro fertilization (IVF) cycles. J Assist Reprod Genet. 1999;16:410-15.

12. Farquhar C, Brown J, Marjoribanks J. Laparoscopic drilling by diathermy or laser for ovulation induction in anovulatory polycystic ovary syndrome. Cochrane Database Syst Rev. 2012;(6):CD001122.

13. Fernandez H, Morin-Surruca M, Torre A, et al. Ovarian drilling for surgical treatment of polycystic ovarian syndrome: a comprehensive review. Reprod Biomed Online. 2011;22:556-68.

14. Marcoux S, Maheux R, Berube S. Laparoscopic surgery in infertile women with minimal or mild endometriosis. Canadian Collaborative Group on Endometriosis. N Engl J Med. 1997;337:217-22.

15. Olive DL, Stohs GF, Metzger DA, et al. Expectant management and hydrotubations in the treatment of endometriosis-associated infertility. Fertil Steril. 1985;44:35-41.

16. Nezhat C, Crowgey S, Nezhat F. Videolaseroscopy for the treatment of endometriosis associated with infertility. Fertil Steril. 1989;51:237-40.

17. Vercellini P, Somigliana E, Vigano P, et al. Surgery for endometriosis-associated infertility: a pragmatic approach. Hum Reprod. 2009;24:254-69.

18. Hart RJ, Hickey M, Maouris P, et al. Excisional surgery versus ablative surgery for ovarian endometriomata. Cochrane Database Syst Rev. 2008;(2):CD004992.

19. Beretta P, Franchi M, Ghezzi F, et al. Randomized clinical trial of two laparoscopic treatments of endometriomas: cystectomy versus drainage and coagulation. Fertil Steril. 1998;70:1176-80.

20. Rickes D, Nickel I, Kropf S, et al. Increased pregnancy rates after ultralong postoperative therapy with gonadotropin-releasing hormone analogs in patients with endometriosis. Fertil Steril. 2002;78(4):757-62.

21. Hammadieh N, Coomarasamy A. Ultrasound-guided hydrosalpinx aspiration during oocyte collection improves pregnancy outcome in IVF: A randomized controlled trial. Hum Reprod. 2008;23:1113-7.

22. Camus E, Poncelet C, Goffinet F, et al. Pregnancy rates after in-vitro fertilization in cases of tubal infertility with and without hydrosalpinx: a meta-analysis of published comparative studies. Hum Reprod. 1999;14(5):1243-9.

23. Zeyneloglu HB, Arici A, Olive DL. Adverse effects of hydrosalpinx on pregnancy rates after in vitro fertilization–embryo transfer. Fertil Steril. 1998;70(3):492-9.

24. Johnson NP, Mak W, Sowter MC. Laparoscopic salpingectomy for women with hydrosalpinges enhances the success of IVF: a Cochrane review. Hum Reprod. 2002;17(3):543-8.

25. Mahran A, Ibrahim M, Bahaa H. The effect of endometrial injury on first cycle IVF/ICSI outcome: a randomized controlled trial. Int J Reprod Biomed (Yazd). 2016;14:193-8.

26. Nastri CO, Lensen SF, Gibreel A, et al. Endometrial injury in women undergoing assisted reproductive techniques. Cochrane Database Syst Rev. 2015;3:CD009517.

27. Shahrokh-Tehraninejad E, Dashti M, Hossein-Rashidi B, et al. A randomized trial to evaluate the effect of local endometrial injury on the clinical pregnancy rate of frozen embryo transfer cycles in patients with repeated implantation failure. J Family Reprod Health. 2016;10:108-14.

Index

Page numbers followed by *f* refer to figure, and *t* refer to table

Gonadotropin-releasing hormone 1, 8, 18, 23, 53, 63
  agonist 32, 33
Granulocyte colony stimulating factor 6, 29, 32, 34
  intrauterine perfusion of 26
Granulocyte-macrophage colony-stimulating factor 40
Granulosa cells 6
Growth hormone 1, 3, 5, 6, 23, 32, 35, 50, 52
  releasing
    factor 6
    hormones 23

H

Heparin 2, 3, 5, 10, 28, 32, 33
  mechanism of action of 28*f*
Homeostatic model assessment 19
Human chorionic gonadotropin 5, 23, 29, 32, 33, 50, 52, 56
  low-dose 26, 29
Human fertilization and embryology authority 40, 46
Human menopausal gonadotropin 8
Human oocytes activation 41
Human serum albumin 40
Hyaluronan-enriched transfer medium 40
Hyaluronic acid 39
Hyaluronic binding assay score 39
Hydrosalpinx 68
  bilateral 68*f*
  disconnection of 6
  removal of 6
Hydroxyvitamin D 19
Hyperinsulinemia 8
Hyperthyroid 53
Hypnosis 5, 11
Hypomenorrhea 65
Hypothesis 45
Hypothyroid 53
Hypothyroidism, subclinical 56, 59
Hysterosalpingography, abnormal 11
Hysteroscopic myomectomy 62, 63
  complications of 63
Hysteroscopic surgeries, postoperative management in 65

I

Immune therapy 2, 5
Immunoglobulin 10
  A 10
  G 10
Implantation 59, 60
  failure, recurrent 10, 63
  rate 32
In vitro fertilization 3, 5, 32
  additional therapy in 1
  outcome 6, 11

program 5
  treatment 1, 5, 18, 23, 28, 37, 59, 62, 64, 67
Infertility 62, 65
  globally, prevalence of 37
  history of 64
  severe male factor 38
Injury, endometrial 3
Inositol 8, 9, 18
Insulin
  growth factor 1 18, 23, 28, 29, 41
  resistance 8
  sensitizing agents 18
International Committee for Monitoring Assisted Reproductive Technology 37
International Federation of Gynecology and Obstetrics Classification 63
International Societies, guidelines of 59*t*
Intracytoplasmic morphologically selected sperm injection 12, 13, 37, 38*f*, 46
Intracytoplasmic sperm injection 1, 2, 7, 23, 29, 32, 37, 58
Intralipid 10
Intramural fibroids 63
Intrauterine granulocyte-colony stimulating factor instillation 29
Intrauterine insemination 67
  cycles 27
Ions 40

K

Ketoconazole 8

L

L-arginine 5, 7, 26, 28, 32, 33
Laser-assisted zona hatching technology 44
Letrozole 8, 53
Leukemia inhibiting factor 59
Levothyroxine 58, 59
Leydig cells 52, 53
Lipids 40
Lipoic acid 20
Live birth rate 6, 32, 37
L-methylfolate 8, 9
Low molecular weight heparin 26, 28
  inhibits 2
Luteal phase
  adjuvants for 32
  estradiol in 24
Luteinizing hormone 6, 18, 23, 27, 57, 66
  recombinant 23
  therapy 52
Lycopene 52

M

Magnesium 19
Massage therapy 11

Matrix metalloproteinase 59
Meiotic spindle 42*f*
Melatonin 3, 5, 8, 9
Methylprednisolone 5, 8
Methylxanthine 33
Metroplasty, hysteroscopic lateral 64
Micronutrients 5, 11
Mid-tubal block 62
Miscarriage
  idiopathic recurrent 2
  recurrent 45
Mitochondrial deoxyribonucleic acid 41
  load measurement 41
Mitochondrial function 41
Morcellator, hysteroscopic 63
Müllerian anomalies 64
Myoinositol 5
Myomas 63
Myomectomy, laparoscopic 62, 63
Myometrium 27

N

N-acetylcysteine 5, 8, 9, 19, 50
Natural killer cell 2, 10, 27, 34
Neuromuscular electric stimulation 34
Nimodipine 27
Nitric oxide donor 33
Nonpharmacological adjuvants 5, 11

O

Obesity 53
Omega-3 fatty acids 20
Oocyte 42*f*, 59, 60
  matured in vitro, fertilization of 2
  meiotic stage, assessment of 42*f*
Ovarian
  drilling, laparoscopic 6, 62, 66
  endometrioma, management of 6
  follicle 57
  hyperstimulation
    function 58
    syndrome 7, 10, 66
  response 22
  stimulation 14, 59
Ovulation 59, 60
Ovum pick-up 29
Oxidative stress 11

P

Pelvic floor neuromuscular electrical stimulation 30, 34
Pentoxifylline 26, 28, 32, 33, 51
Phosphodiesterase type 5 27
Physiological intracytoplasmic sperm injection 12, 13, 37, 39, 46
Pituitary downregulation 14
Placentation 59, 60
Platelet
  derived growth factor 29
  rich plasma 26, 29, 32, 35

EU GSPR Authorised Reprsentative
Logos Europe, 9 rue Nicolas Poussin
1700, La Rochelle, France
Phone: +33 (0) 6 67 93 73 78
E-mail: contact@logoseurope.eu